BEAT CELLULITE NOW

10 Steps To Banish Cellulite Forever

Liz Hodgkinson

Thorsons

Thorsons

An Imprint of HarperCollins*Publishers*

77–85 Fulham Palace Road,

Hammersmith, London W6 8JB

The Thorsons website address is: www.Thorsons.com

Based on *The Anti-Cellulite Plan* published by Thorsons 1990, 1992

Published by Thorsons 2000

10 9 8 7 6 5 4 3 2 1

Liz Hodgkinson asserts the moral right to
be identified as the author of this work

A catalogue record for this book
is available from the British Library

ISBN 0 7225 3978 9

Printed and bound in Great Britain by

Woolnough Bookbinding Ltd,

Irthlingborough, Northamptonshire

BEAT
CELLULITE
NOW

Contents

Acknowledgements

I should particularly like to thank aromatherapists Patricia Davis and Frances Clifford for expert help in preparing this book. Thanks are also due to nutritionist Celia Wright, who first opened my eyes to the problem of cellulite, and to masseuse Clare Maxwell-Hudson, for valuable information on the many benefits of massage.

Introduction
The Curse of Eve

Around 80 per cent of women in the Western world suffer from cellulite. The good news is that cellulite is not an unavoidable curse of Eve – it is treatable and removable.

Interestingly, it is only in recent years that the existence of cellulite has been recognized by the orthodox medical profession. For a long time, doctors in Britain and America were extremely scornful of the whole idea of cellulite which they firmly believed was simply another way that get-rich-quick cosmetic companies were conning vain, credulous women. Even though they could not deny the observable fact that many women had lumps and bumps on their thighs, there was no real evidence, they maintained, to suggest that cellulite existed as a separate entity to, or was in any way different from, ordinary fat.

Alternative practitioners, on the other hand, had always maintained that cellulite did exist. But until the alternative medicine revolution of the eighties, these practitioners were held in low esteem by the medical profession.

In France, the story is very different. Over there, cellulite has been accepted as a genuine medical condition for the past forty years. So much do they accept its existence that you can have anti-cellulite treatments on their equivalent of the National Health Service.

Now the tide is turning in Britain and America and although it would not be true to say that every single doctor accepts the existence of cellulite, at least *some* medically-qualified people now believe that the evidence for its reality has become overwhelming.

WHAT IS CELLULITE?

Cellulite is the popular name given to those peculiarly female bulges which collect on thighs, buttocks and upper arms and which go into 'orange-peel' puckers when pressed and squeezed. The cellulite areas feel cold to the touch since circulation is poor in those areas. You will also find that the skin on cellulite areas is whiter and more difficult to tan than other skin.

The bulges are in fact fat cells that have become filled with waterlogged toxic deposits, caused mainly by eating the wrong kinds of foods and living the wrong kind of lifestyle.

The presence of cellulite is nothing to do with being over-weight. You can be verging on anorexia and still have cellulite deposits. Conversely, you can be extremely fat and not have any cellulite.

HOW DO WE GET CELLULITE AND WHY?

Cellulite is a problem confined to women. Men never get it. It is widely accepted that there is a hormonal factor involved. The condition is caused, above all, by the presence of oestrogen. The more oestrogen there is in a woman's body, the more likely it is that cellulite will develop. The danger times for developing cellulite are at puberty, pregnancy and the menopause, the times of greatest hormonal fluctuation.

Unless women are frequently pregnant, they have high levels of oestrogen circulating around their system continuously. The amount of oestrogen circulating in women's bodies has also increased enormously since the mid 1960s with the introduction of the contraceptive pill and hormone replacement therapy.

Oestrogen has a specific purpose and that is to prepare the body to receive and nurture an embryo. Whenever pregnancy occurs, the amount of oestrogen circulating in the system drops rapidly. Nowadays most women have far more oestrogen circulating in their system than was intended by nature. It acts to send waste materials away from vital organs and into areas where they will be relatively harmless. This eventually becomes apparent as cellulite. In men, waste products have the effect of furring up their arteries so they are more likely to succumb to heart attacks. It seems as if biology acts to protect the female. We get cellulite whereas men get hardening of the arteries – a condition which is taken extremely seriously by most doctors.

In fact, cellulite and heart disease are manifestations of an identical problem – too much stress, a bad diet, too little exercise and too much rubbish getting into the system and not being able to get out.

Another factor, most probably linked to hormones, is that women's bodies simply cannot take the same amount of punishment and abuse that men's can. We know now for a fact that women's tolerance threshold for alcohol and nicotine is far lower than men's. But all the time women are abusing their bodies, oestrogen performs its powerful protective function and does its best to send the waste to outlying areas so that we will survive.

Finally, latest research shows that cellulite is the gradual accumulation of fluid and toxic matter in the connective tissues. When cellulite starts to accumulate, the connective tissues in the fat cells are irritated and begin to harden. The effect of this is to compress the blood vessels, cutting off circulation and preventing the normal biological processes, such as the operation of the lymphatic system, from doing their jobs of eliminating the unwanted materials. Instead of being carried away as they should, the fluid and toxic matter continue to build up around the connective tissues. These migrate to the dermis where they remain and harden. The result is the dreaded 'orange peel' skin.

If the mass is merely fat, as opposed to cellulite, say the researchers, the skin remains smooth. Fat by itself will never cause the lumpy, bumpy appearance characteristic of cellulite. The difference between obesity and cellulite is that with the former the fatty cells can move freely; they are not blocked. With cellulite, by contrast, the fat cells are trapped in connective tissue, and this is why cellulite-laden areas feel hard and knobbly, not soft like ordinary fat areas.

Although cellulite is not exactly fat, it is caused by a serious malfunction of the fat cells. One reason why women are prone to this condition rather than men is that women have twice the amount of fatty tissue of men, and the ability of their fat cells to multiply is twice as great. There is also far more connective tissue in women's bodies.

To sum up, cellulite forms when there is a general circulatory problem in the body. It is, above all, an indication of a sluggish circulation, a sign that body wastes cannot be disposed of in the normal way. When cellulite is present, this means that the lymphatic system, the body's main vacuum cleaner, cannot do its job, and there is internal clogging.

The next step is to understand what causes the clogging in the first place.

THE MAIN CAUSES OF CELLULITE

Cellulite forms when women's bodies produce or take in too much oestrogen, resulting in waste matter being pushed away from vital organs. But oestrogen will not send rubbish to outlying areas unless there is rubbish to send. So the first thing to understand about cellulite is that it is caused mainly by leading the wrong lifestyle, such as:

1 **the wrong kind of diet**

2 **too much caffeine, alcohol and nicotine**

3 **stress**

4 **a sedentary lifestyle**

Although cellulite has probably always existed, the problem is getting worse. The main reason for this is that more women than ever smoke, drink, eat processed foods and take prescription drugs such as the pill.

ARE THERE DIFFERENT TYPES OF CELLULITE?

Recently, researchers have identified two distinct types of cellulite: the type that sits on the surface and the 'stubborn' cellulite which is much further down and which takes more effort to encourage to disappear.

Skin specialist, Sally Gilbert Wilson, believes that cellulite can be categorized in several ways.

There is the predominantly DIETARY kind of cellulite which is associated with a high-fat diet. This type of cellulite is easy to cure because it responds well to the anti-cellulite diet.

The METABOLIC type of cellulite is common in slim people and is caused mainly by sluggish metabolism and a sedentary job. Skin brushing to detoxify and the anti-cellulite diet are usually enough to shift toxic matter caused in this way.

The mainly HORMONAL kind of cellulite is found on women who suffer from PMT, post-natal depression or who have problems with the pill. Deep connective tissue massage is the best solution here.

According to Sally, the worst kind of cellulite, and the hardest to shift, is the INHERITED KIND. If your sisters, mother, grandmother or female relatives suffered from cellulite, then do not exactly abandon hope – but expect the struggle to be a prolonged one. Aromatherapy combined with skin brushing to improve circulation provides the best form of attack.

MY STORY

I had been plagued by lumpy, bumpy, blancmange thighs for most of my adult life. Over the years I tried everything I could to get rid of the bulges and regain the slim, shapely thighs of my pre-adolescence. I went on stringent diets. I did huge amounts of exercise. I went to health farms and submitted myself to saunas, starvation regimes and endless pummelling and pounding.

While this effort ensured that I became extremely thin everywhere else, the thigh bulges stayed firmly in place, apparently unbudgeable.

Eventually, I heard about a treatment which was actually guaranteed to get rid of cellulite. I decided to give it a try. The treatment consisted of a combination of a detoxifying diet, brushing yourself with a hard, scratchy brush made of Mexican cactus, and having aromatherapy oil massaged into the bulges. A few weeks of this regime, I was assured, would make my cellulite go away.

Well, all I can say is that the treatments did work – wonderfully. Nobody was more surprised than I when the lumps and bumps which had been there for two decades, seemingly unshiftable, finally began to soften and eventually disappear altogether. The deposits were simply waste material that for a long time I hadn't been able to get rid of – and now I had succeeded.

THE ANTI-CELLULITE PLAN: 10 STEPS TO BANISH CELLULITE FOREVER

The cellulite cure outlined in this book is not a treatment worked out by medical doctors. It has been developed over the years by nutritionists, aromatherapists and masseurs – and it is guaranteed to work. There are no adverse side effects, no harsh drugs to take and no danger.

It consists of four main elements: diet, dry skin brushing, aromatherapy and massage. All of these four ingredients are absolutely essential in any effective cellulite-banishing regime. Other elements, such as exercise, are highly recommended but optional extras.

With its simple, step-by-step approach, this book offers advice about the latest treatments available – such as the new herbal pill Cellasene – and shows how a combination of the right diet, body brushing, massage and the correct essential oils means that cellulite can be completely eradicated forever.

HOW DO I BEGIN?

The best way to begin is gradually. Although the plan is extremely beneficial to health generally, it has to be realized that a toxic body takes time to heal itself. The more toxic the system is, the longer any cleansing plan will take.

Also the body may react unfavourably at first to a drastic change in diet, however healthy this diet may be. We are primarily creatures of habit, and our bodies get used to whatever foods and drinks we give them. They may rebel when anything is withdrawn suddenly.

If you smoke, drink a lot of alcohol, eat junk foods, down several cups of coffee a day, and are also extremely sedentary, it is unrealistic to suppose that you can revert to good habits in a single day. You will not be able to give up all your props and addictions at once as this will represent too drastic a change for your system to handle. Also, you may well feel extremely deprived and as if life is not worth living. It is only when people become released from their addictions and cravings that they come to realize that life is actually *more* enjoyable without the artificial props.

Before you embark on the anti-cellulite diet (see Step 4) you really need to give up smoking, tea and coffee. The first two weeks of the diet are really strict and no caffeine or nicotine is allowed.

After those gruelling two weeks, the diet is modified and you are even allowed the occasional cup of tea and coffee.

Once you start the diet you can consider that you have started the anti-cellulite regime proper. At the same time as beginning the diet, do the body brushing (see Step 6) and use essential oils for massage (see Steps 7 and 8).

HOW LONG BEFORE THE CELLULITE STARTS TO GO?

This depends on how strict you are with yourself and how much cellulite you have in the first place.

Most therapists reckon that six treatments – if possible – two a week combined with diet and brushing at home will rid thighs of cellulite. In my own case it took far longer, but then I had suffered severe cellulite for two decades.

Before starting, measure your thighs at the thickest part and note down the measurement. Then, as you proceed with the plan, measure your thighs weekly to see if there is any difference. There will certainly be a measurable loss after about a month.

If after two weeks you don't seem to be getting anywhere, don't give up hope. There is no cellulite in the world that can withstand the regime detailed in this book – so long as you follow it conscientiously and regularly. It is the *regularity of the treatments which does the trick. Nothing will work if it is remembered only occasionally.*

THE ANTI-CELLULITE PLAN

PRE-PLAN		PLAN
Cut Out	*Cut Down*	*Take Up*
Smoking	Alcohol	Detoxifying diet for two weeks
	Coffee	Dry skin brushing daily *before* bath
		Massage using aromatherapy oils *after* bath

POST-PLAN

Keep Up
Exercise for toning
Healthy diet
Skin brushing twice a week
Occasional massage

STEP 1

ANTI-CELLULITE CREAMS AND HERBAL PILLS
Buy them – or bin them?

ANTI-CELLULITE CREAMS

When anti-cellulite creams first came on the market in the mid-seventies I was highly sceptical of them. I wanted to believe the claims made by the manufacturers of these creams but common sense seemed to tell me that they couldn't possibly work. It appeared most likely they belonged in exactly the same category as hair-restorers, bust enlargers and pills to restore sexual potency and attractiveness. In other words, they were preying on universal fears ripe for exploitation by the get-rich-quick merchants since the beginning of time.

The products did not seem to even begin to work. Those of us who tried them found that however hard we rubbed them in, the lumps and bumps remained as firmly in place as ever.

Before long, the Advertising and Standards Authority stepped in to say that the claims made for the creams and lotions were unsupported by any scientific evidence and should be withdrawn. As a result, the claims that these products could magically melt away fat, themselves melted away, and were replaced by more innocuous wording such as 'improve circulation'. Well, you couldn't argue about the ability of a cream to improve circulation if you rubbed it in vigorously enough. Most of these products stayed on the market, however, although sales must have been adversely affected.

Today, there are very many creams available, with more coming out all the time. I have somewhat revised my opinion of them since they first came on the market – mainly because I now know so much more about cellulite than I did then.

Do they work?

Most of the creams and lotions containing the results of the 'latest scientific research' are extremely expensive. But do they work?

I now believe that some patent creams can work. But *I will only believe the claims of patent products where these are backed up by serious research carried out in hospitals by proper, independent doctors – and have published papers on their results.*

Many anti-cellulite preparations are riding on the backs of the companies who have carried out proper research and have investigated the subject seriously. This means that a large number of the companies manufacturing anti-cellulite treatments have not carried out their own proper research into the subject.

I also believe that the creams will only work so long as the massage is kept up daily for at least a month. I also believe that expensive creams work better *after* the cellulite has been attacked by aromatherapy, and if possible, professional lymphatic drainage massage. Also there is diet – don't forget that. It is most important and means that the cellulite has at least a chance of disappearing forever. There can only be, at best, a modest difference when creams and lotions are applied and there is no attempt made to follow the anti-cellulite diet. Otherwise, as fast as you are sculpturing your body with the aid of the scientifically-developed cream, you are encouraging new bulges and lumps to form by eating the wrong food. So you will be fighting a losing battle.

> **An effective anti-cellulite regime must start with diet in order to attack the problem from inside out rather than outside in.**

How Can I Tell If My Cream is Working?

You can tell if your cream is working by taking measurements and noticing the frequency of urination. When cellulite starts to shift, the very first thing you notice is that you want to pee every hour on the hour. The other unmistakable sign is that the bulges and indentations start to smooth out and also you lose that cold, clammy feeling.

It is, though, notoriously difficult to know for sure whether such and such a heavily-advertised cream might be working, or whether one is being over-optimistic or influenced by wishful thinking. Beauty and health magazines which ask readers to be guinea pigs and try certain treatments for a month or so find that reports back are rarely positive. Readers almost always say that the products have made no difference whatever and that their lumps and bumps are as firmly in place as ever.

Cheap Versus Expensive

Which? magazine recently tested a whole series of patent anti-cellulite products to see whether they made any difference. They also asked a number of volunteers to test cheap creams – the thing about most anti-cellulite products is that they are extremely expensive.

The *Which?* researchers came to the conclusion that the cheap creams worked just as well as the expensive imported products BUT – and this is an important but – they came to the conclusion that daily application and dedicated massage does indeed make a difference. Cellulite deposits definitely disappeared with diligent, regular massage.

Buy them – or Bin Them?

Whatever cream, oil or lotion you buy, you will be wasting your money completely *unless* you are also prepared to go on a diet and undertake daily body brushing. Remember that with any anti-cellulite regime, even if you go to a clinic which specializes in anti-cellulite treatments, 60 per cent of the work has to come from you.

Even though some of the creams do work, it is far better to use essential oils than cream (see Step 7) as they penetrate deeper down into the skin and have an effect on the whole system. For thousands of years, Indian ayurvedic medicine has known that herbal oils have a dramatic detoxifying effect, something that not even the most expensive cream can achieve.

As aromatherapist Frances Clifford says, you can't stop essential oils from working, whereas creams will stay on the surface.

THE NEW HERBAL PILLS

Cellasene

Of course, all cellulite sufferers are looking for a painless, diet-free, exercise-free method of ridding themselves of ghastly bumps and lumps, and a new development in anti-cellulite creams has come to their aid. Many years' medical research into the causes of cellulite has resulted in the manufacture of a herbal pill, Cellasene, which is formulated to attack cellulite from the inside. Said to work by repairing the arteries, veins and circulation in the areas affected by cellulite, the pills are also designed to help increase the metabolic rate to break down fatty deposits in the affected areas.

All you do is take two pills a day for eight weeks – and be astonished at the difference. Clinical trials on Cellasene have certainly been very impressive, and at least show that the problem is now starting to be taken seriously by doctors, instead of dismissed as nonsense. Since Cellasene arrived on the market in 1998, a number of other manufacturers have also produced herbal pills designed to eliminate toxic deposits from fatty cells.

Buy Them – or Bin Them?

Only time will tell whether these new formations are a genuine breakthrough, or whether they will eventually go the way of most other patent anti-cellulite treatments.

OTHER TREATMENTS

A form of treatment which has become popular in France, although it has hardly caught on in the UK yet, is **mesotherapy**, where cellulite-laden areas are pricked with a series of tiny needles which penetrate the area with anti-cellulite oils. Apparently, it doesn't hurt and it should certainly work.

Normaform is a form of lymphatic drainage which is used in beauty salons and health farms to get rid of cellulite. Basically the equipment consists of a pair of inflatable leggings which look like enormous Wellington boots. The leggings are inflated to fit the legs very tightly and constitute a form of massage. The air pressure is designed to improve the natural circulation of the blood and tissue fluids through stimulation of the lymph flow. The idea is that the treatment will rid the body of water retention.

The treatment is quite painless, although it feels rather strange, and after an hour's treatment, when the leggings are taken off, you will notice a network of tiny white lines up and down your legs. This is where the lymph channels have been raised and the lines will go down in about an hour. No harm results from this treatment.

The equipment works to speed up the flow of lymph in much the same way as vigorous exercise and helps to rid tissues of waste product. About six treatments would be necessary to rid the legs of cellulite deposits. Again, this form of treatment is best combined with the anti-cellulite diet otherwise the cellulite will just come back.

Most health farms and beauty clinics now offer a whole range of passive treatments for cellulite such as **ionithermie** – thermal clay treatments where you are smeared with a thick green substance then an electrical current embeds the active ingredients deep into the tissues – and **toning tables** designed to give you isometric exercises. The trouble with these is that one application, or even treatments over a period of time, won't make the slightest bit of difference. Many people book themselves in for a week at a health farm and are then disappointed because in spite of starving themselves, having loads of treatments and electrical currents passed through them, and so on, the cellulite is just as firmly in place at the end of their stay.

This doesn't mean the treatments are not any good. A week simply isn't long enough to make any noticeable difference to the cellulite deposits. Few people are aware of any improvement before a period of a month, at least.

REMEMBER. There is *no* way of escaping the diet! All expensive creams and patent treatments, plus visits to the beauty therapist, will certainly help but around 60 per cent of the effort has to come from *you*. In spite of ever-more sophisticated treatments to separate you from your cellulite (and your money), nothing will work in the long-term unless you adhere to the diet.

STEP 2
THE USUAL SUSPECTS
The three dietary don'ts – coffee, alcohol and cigarettes

Of all the cellulite-causing substances, the three main culprits are coffee, alcohol and nicotine. If you want to get rid of your ugly lumps and bumps for good, you need to cut out, or at the very least, cut down on coffee, alcohol and cigarettes.

COFFEE

Coffee is probably the most harmful cellulite-causing substance because of the caffeine it contains. The bad effects of coffee have now been well-documented and several medical studies have suggested that **more than three cups a day can do damage**. None of these studies mentions cellulite as a possible adverse side effect of caffeine, but the substance has definitely been linked with all kinds of female complaints from benign breast lumps to pelvic disorders. Caffeine interferes with the uptake of certain minerals in the diet, particularly iron, and also predisposes to certain anxiety states.

The main reason for this is that caffeine puts extra stress on the adrenal glands, which release adrenaline. Like cocaine, caffeine gives the system an instant boost by making the adrenals pump out extra adrenaline. The problem is that when we drink huge amounts of coffee, we enable large quantities of adrenaline to be released which are not burned up at all. Biologically, adrenaline exists to protect us from danger, to enable us to run away or to stay and fight. We naturally get surges of adrenaline when there is a near miss on the motorway, when we are about to sit an important exam or attend a vital interview. Then, when the danger is past, the adrenaline process ceases. Caffeine enables this hormone to be secreted all the time.

So coffee puts extra stress on the adrenals by over-working them. They discharge too much adrenaline into the system and become exhausted. Too much caffeine in the system also puts extra stress onto the kidneys, where all water-soluble rubbish is taken so that the blood can be cleansed.

It is now well-known that a high intake of caffeine puts people at extra risk of heart attack as it increases the amount of cholesterol in the system. This causes even more clogging up. In women, the net result of over-consumption is to increase the amount of cellulite on the thighs. For most women, the presence of cellulite is a potent indicator that they are drinking too much caffeine in the form of tea, coffee or colas. Chocolate also contains a significant amount of caffeine.

Drinks containing caffeine make you feel good by giving you an instant lift, but this is followed by a nasty low – the well-known withdrawal symptoms. In women who are pregnant or on the pill, caffeine is eliminated particularly slowly, which indicates a hormonal link.

Furthermore, coffee beans are loaded with pesticides which in large quantities can upset the digestive process. There is no particular advantage to drinking tea either, as it contains significant amounts of caffeine, though only half as much as coffee, and in addition, can be loaded with impurities such as copper. Consuming anti-nutrients means that the deposits of cellulite can only get bigger.

> **Coffee and tea have now become our most universal stimulants, and we tend to forget that, delicious though they may be, they are actually non-nutrients, substances the body emphatically does not need for its daily functioning.**

The potentially addictive qualities of tea and coffee are warning signs, or should be. The body develops specific cravings only when its biochemistry has been artificially adapted to accommodate an alien substance. If you give your body just what it needs for proper functioning, cravings and addictions do not develop. Unfortunately in our present society, we have mistaken cravings and addictions for excitement. We appear to thrive on artificial sensual stimulation, forgetting that the human body was not originally designed to cope with these substances. It is hardly surprising if, after time, it cannot cope with the onslaught and starts to rebel.

Of course, not everybody who consumes vast quantities of caffeine will get cellulite any more than every single person who smokes will die of lung cancer. Some systems can withstand large amounts of stimulating beverages, while others can't. The fact is that caffeine significantly adds to the burden of the body.

Cut Down

Many people find that cutting down on, or cutting out tea and coffee, is an incredibly hard thing to do. This is because over the years they have become addicted to them, usually without realizing it.

When attempting to cut out tea and coffee you will soon know if you are addicted. Try going without them for 48 hours and see how you feel when drinking herbal substitutes instead. If you are used to drinking more than three cups of tea or coffee in a single day you will most probably experience quite severe withdrawal symptoms ranging from a feeling of disorientation to bad migraine headaches.

In my case the migraine I suffered from sudden caffeine withdrawal was so bad that I had to go to bed. In addition I felt depressed and miserable. It took about a week for the worst of the symptoms to wear off, but I never really felt well while not drinking any tea or coffee.

In the end, my therapist sympathized and advised me to go back to one cup of real coffee a day, so long as it was made from freshly ground beans that were kept in the freezer to ensure freshness. I did, and instantly my spirits lifted. Now I drink that one delicious, not-to-be-missed cup of coffee a day, and have one cup of Luaka or ordinary tea in the afternoon.

The first two weeks of the anti-cellulite diet are very strict and you are required to give up tea and coffee (see Step 4). After this, the diet can be modified and you can enjoy the occasional cup of tea or coffee.

> **REMEMBER** On an anti-cellulite diet, the coffee you drink must be real, made from freshly ground beans. You should not under any circumstances drink the instant variety as this not only has caffeine added but it is made by a high-tech process which renders it completely artificial.

NICOTINE

Nicotine, like caffeine, is extremely bad for women. It is bad for men as well, but it seems that a woman's system is less able to withstand the poisons released by tobacco in the blood-stream. We have known for 20 years or more that smoking during pregnancy causes low birth-weight babies and, more recently, it has also been linked with malformations and brain damage in embryos.

> Nicotine is one of the most addictive drugs available and one of the hardest to get out of the system.

The first effect of nicotine is that it uses up oxygen, reducing the amount available for use by the cells. It does this by decreasing the efficiency of the lungs. It also affects the haemoglobin – red cells – in the blood. Haemoglobin is the main carrier for oxygen in the blood and picks up the oxygen in the lungs as the blood circulates.

If the oxygen exchange in the blood is less efficient because of nicotine intake, then every cell in the body will receive less oxygen than it should. This factor is extremely relevant to the cellulite problem because, above all, oxygen acts as a powerful stimulator and cleanser for the blood. Body cells cannot function without adequate oxygen any more than we can ourselves. Whenever there is reduced oxygen in the body, cell function is impaired and circulation is adversely affected.

Smoking adds to the amount of toxic wastes that enter the body which means that the system has to work even harder to get rid of them. Nicotine is a powerful pollutant and, like caffeine, it is an anti-nutrient. Its effect is to rob the system of essential substances such as Vitamin C and zinc.

Give Up

Those who smoke should make giving up or cutting down an urgent priority before they embark on the anti-cellulite regime.

The difficulty of giving up smoking should never be underestimated. On the other hand, there is little point in undertaking the diet and body brushing if you continue to smoke 20 or more cigarettes a day.

Many women fear that they will put on weight if they give up smoking. By following the anti-cellulite diet, however, smoking can be given up without any danger at all of unwelcome weight gain.

ALCOHOL

Most women drink alcohol regularly these days.

Women can take far less alcohol than men. One reason for this is that female livers are smaller and able to process less. Another reason is that womens bodies have a higher proportion of fat than men's and alcohol does not enter fat cells. This means that its effect is concentrated into a smaller area and takes longer to be processed by the liver.

Alcohol enters the blood very quickly and instantly alters blood chemistry. It adds to the workload of the liver which can very quickly become overloaded. When alcohol is added to the sum total of non-nutrients entering the body the result is that the liver and kidneys cannot effectively handle the excess waste material. For most people, the eliminative organs have enough to do handling ordinary waste materials produced by the diet. If they have to deal with caffeine, nicotine and alcohol loads as well it is not surprising that they find it hard to cope and that much waste matter simply stays in the system.

Cut Down

The good news about alcohol is that after the first booze-free fortnight of the anti-cellulite diet (see Step 4), you can gradually introduce the occasional drink back into your life.

You should, however, never drink extra-strong lagers, which contain huge amounts of sugars, and ideally you should avoid lager altogether, as well as spirits and fortified wines such as port or sherry. Your system *can* cope with an occasional glass of champagne or wine, especially if it is organic. Wines with additives, such as sugar and chemicals, may not do the system any good, but the organic ones can actually help digestion. When drinking champagne, intersperse it with non-fizzy mineral water. If you drink the sparkling kind, you will accumulate too much gas and bloating will result.

STEP 3
WATER OF LIFE
Drink at least a litre a day

These days, most people do not drink enough water. In fact, most of us are chronically dehydrated and this dehydration contributes to cellulite deposits being laid down – and staying there – because they cannot get out of a system which has become sluggish like a pond full of weeds. Water moves rubbish as well as nutrients through the system and we need to keep our own internal waterways clear and unclogged. The way to do this is to keep water driving through the system.

Very many people never drink any water at all and imagine that diet colas, fruit juices and 'health drinks' do much the same job.

In fact, water is the only drink that can successfully rehydrate the body and help to flush out toxins and accumulated wastes from the system. *No other drink can do this.* Whenever you have a drink which is not water, award it minus points, and make sure you have a glass of water to compensate for it. Remember, nothing which is not water counts as water even though all drinks *contain* water.

HOW MUCH SHOULD I DRINK?

You should drink at least a litre of water a day to rehydrate and detoxify the body.

If you find it difficult, as many people do at first, try to get into the habit of having a big glass of water by your side all day long. This is especially important if you work in a modern office. Drink a glass of water before you go to bed, and drink a glass first thing in the morning before you have anything else to drink. As buying water can become expensive, try drinking plain, boiled, cooled water. If you can drink it warm, it is kinder to the system than ice-cold water.

If you buy mineral water, any brand on the market will do. In my case I found constant Perrier and Badoit so boring that I kept forgetting to drink them. For me, the carbonated drinks are slightly more interesting and fun to drink than the still ones, although not much.

> **TIP** Boiling water is just as effective as filtering it and avoids the bother and expense of water filters. Also, if you fill a plastic bottle of water from the tap and leave it overnight in the fridge, the calcium will dissolve and the water will taste almost indistinguishable from mineral water. We've almost come to believe that tap water is poisonous but the problem is that if you always drink bought water, you may imagine you have no drinkable stuff when you run out.

A FINAL WORD

When people first start drinking more water, they often feel sick. This is because their bodies are having to get used to taking in more and have become unaccustomed to it. If you feel sick when drinking extra water, don't gulp it down, but sip it slowly.

STEP 4
YOU ARE WHAT YOU EAT
Time for a detox

The right diet, dry skin brushing, aromatherapy and massage are the four most important steps in your war against cellulite. All these four ingredients are absolutely essential in any anti-cellulite regime, but most vital is diet. Because even if you manage to get rid of some cellulite with oils and massage, it will always come back unless you can prevent more forming with the correct diet.

The anti-cellulite diet does two main jobs: it cleanses and detoxifies the whole system to enable toxic wastes to be eliminated and it prevents more cellulite from forming in the future.

WHY THE MODERN DIET IS SO BAD

Although deposits of cellulite can be seen clearly in the paintings of Rubens, Rembrandt and Renoir, it is unlikely that women living in pre-literate societies ever collected much of the stuff. In fact, very few women living what we might call a 'natural' life – eating whole foods, lots of fruit and vegetables and not drinking tea, coffee or alcohol – ever develop a cellulite problem.

In the modern West, the eliminative difficulties caused by smoking, coffee and alcohol consumption are exacerbated by an artificial diet.

When a pure natural diet is eaten, the liver and large intestine are extremely efficient at getting rid of wastes very quickly. In fact, the more natural the food, the quicker the digestive system breaks it down. The more artificial it becomes, the longer it takes to go through the body. In some cases, the artificial substance may not be eliminated by the body at all and may simply stay in the system, sometimes for years on end.

Much of the waste material that is not handled by the liver or large intestine gets reabsorbed back into the body where it starts to do damage. It is when too much waste material accumulates that we notice cellulite deposits. The more the system is clogged up and the more sluggish circulation becomes, the worse the cellulite problem is likely to be.

Cellulite-encouraging foodstuffs are sugar, dairy produce, meat and anything processed, smoked or preserved. Sugar has a similar effect on the body to caffeine in that it releases adrenalin and gives a quick energy boost, followed by a 'down' not long after. Dairy produce is mucus-forming, which means that it encourages waste material to become sticky and stay in the system. Meat products also take a long time to be processed by the body and, in some cases, may never be entirely eliminated.

THE ANTI-CELLULITE DIET

All restricted food-intake diets are tough and the anti-cellulite diet is no exception. But for anyone who really wants to get rid of the lumps and bumps it's not an optional extra but an absolute necessity.

So there's nothing for it but to make up your mind to become spartan and abstemious, at least until the cellulite has gone away.

The diet advocated here is the one first developed by Dr Weston

Price, a dentist who went round the world recording the diet of people in pre-literate societies. He discovered time and again that the closer to nature their food, the healthier they stayed. The 'primitive' diets eaten by these people appeared to be the real key to their continuing good health. From this Dr Price concluded that the more removed from nature a diet was, the worse the general health of any community became. The more people ate white bread, chips, salted peanuts, crisps and processed foods, the more they suffered from ill-health.

Over the years, Dr Price's ideas were taken up by other doctors and nutritionists who, until the 1980s, remained mainly on the fringes and were considered extremely cranky and peculiar. It wasn't until people such as health writer Leslie Kenton, nutritionists Celia Wright and Patrick Holford, and Dr Alan Stewart of the British Society for Nutritional Medicine, began writing about these diets in popular magazines that they gained general acceptance.

I say 'acceptance' but of course, the 'healthy' diet still is not accepted by everybody as the main ingredient of lasting health. Some authorities still laugh at the idea of 'detoxifying' and clearing the system of poisons by a pure diet. But the monastic, detoxifying diet is what health farms all over the world have been advocating for the past hundred years at least, and it has proven highly effective in getting rid of cellulite.

CLEANSE YOUR SYSTEM – THE TWO-WEEK DETOXIFYING DIET

When embarking on an anti-cellulite regime, it is essential to cleanse and detoxify the system from inside first. So you must begin with a very strict two-week cleansing and detoxifying diet.

What Can I Drink?

As mentioned in Step 2, you really have to cut out tea and coffee, ideally drinking neither for at least two weeks. It is also important to avoid all alcohol, if possible, when on the initial cleansing diet.

At the same time as cutting down on tea and coffee, it is important to increase considerably your intake of mineral water. When starting the cleansing regime, you should drink as many as eight glasses of mineral water a day.

Fruit juices can be drunk in moderation, and preferably diluted with mineral water as 'neat' they can be too strong for a system in the process of detoxification. Of course, avoid all sugar-laden fruit drinks and squashes.

What Can I Eat?

Now we come to the thorny subject of food. Ideally, all your food should be raw, organically grown, eaten on the day of purchase, or picked from your own garden, unfrozen, unprocessed, unsalted, untreated in any way. Clearly this kind of diet is virtually impossible for anybody to follow at home, although some health farms specialize in this kind of therapy.

For the important two weeks of your cleansing regime you should try to eat nothing but fruit and vegetables. The main idea behind the **fruit-and-vegetable-only** diet is that these are the foods the body finds easiest to digest. They will not put any strain on the liver or kidneys. The more difficult foods are to digest, the less chance you will have of the cellulite disappearing. You can't expect the organs of elimination to be able to do everything at once. Anything processed, cooked or generally denatured adds to the burden of the digestive system.

But don't imagine that any old fruit and vegetables will do. Far from it. Even here you have to be careful. Citrus fruits such as oranges and grapefruit are out except very occasionally, as they are rather rough on the liver. But definitely in are bananas, apples, pears, pineapple, all the exotica such as mangoes, papaya, passion fruit, kiwi fruit, grapes, strawberries, raspberries and blackberries.

Good vegetables are: potatoes, spinach, cauliflower, broccoli, cabbage, mange tout, beans, turnips, swedes, green peppers, carrots and celery. Not all of these can be eaten raw, of course, but wherever possible, eat without cooking. Spinach, cauliflower and broccoli are delicious raw with a small amount of vinaigrette or lemon dressing.

HOW WILL I FEEL?

Some people say they feel wonderful straight away on an all-fruit-and-vegetable diet. Many more will feel quite terrible at first. This is mainly because the body takes time to adapt to any radical change of diet. So you should be prepared for some feelings of disorientation and discomfort, for cravings, depression and bad temper. These are withdrawal symptoms, a sign that something is happening and they won't last for more than a few days.

In addition you will certainly find changes in bowel movements and frequency of urination. You may also find that you sweat more and you may erupt in the kind of spots you haven't had since adolescence. Some women also experience menstrual changes or suffer from insomnia.

None of these symptoms is anything to worry about – they are simply indications that the body is at last getting rid of toxic waste. To add insult to injury, it is extremely unlikely that you will notice any difference in the cellulite at first. It will usually be a week or two before the stuff even begins to shift.

> **TIP:** When starting the anti-cellulite diet you have to give priority to this form of eating. It's not a good idea to do it at the same time as moving house, starting a new job, or undergoing any emotional or physical upheavals. Getting rid of cellulite is hard work and upheaval enough, and you should, ideally, concentrate on this task alone for a time.

WHAT CAN I EAT AND DRINK IN A TYPICAL DAY?

Here is a typical day's eating and drinking plan for the first two weeks on an anti-cellulite regime.

ON RISING

A glass of hot water with a small amount of lemon, or one of the 'wake-up' herb teas such as Early Morn, or a glass of cold water. Always use mineral rather than tap water for early morning drinks if you can.

BREAKFAST

A couple of bananas, apples or a huge bunch of grapes. That's it. Plus, of course, mineral water either half an hour before or half an hour after the fruit. Most nutritional experts do not advise eating or drinking together as water dilutes the digestive juices.

Those who know that they are simply not going to be able to manage on fruit alone should not reach for the nearest slice of bread but should nibble sunflower, sesame or pumpkin seeds. If you have a coffee grinder, grind up equal amounts of these seeds and sprinkle them on the fruit. Then you won't feel hungry although it may be difficult at first not to eat that really delicious toast, butter and marmalade that the others are tucking into.

MID-MORNING

Eat more fruit if you are at home. If at work, take a selection of fruit and seeds with you. Bananas are particularly good at assuaging hunger.

LUNCH

Whenever possible, eat a large salad consisting of raw vegetables. Carrots, cauliflower and broccoli are all quite filling and you can eat as much of them as you like. Those who are not used to raw vegetables may find eating them very odd at first, although they are becoming more accepted nowadays.

You can now buy juicers which are well worth the outlay to have fresh fruit and vegetable juices throughout the day.

Note: If you are avoiding dairy products, as you should be, it is a good idea to take a calcium supplement.

MID-AFTERNOON

Have a cup of herb tea if you are feeling like crawling up the wall by now, and some more fruit. Throughout the day, drink lots of mineral water, but not too many herb teas. Some of them can be quite strong.

SUPPER

Here you can have some vegetable soup sprinkled with ground seeds, and then another huge vegetable salad, or just some more fruit if you can manage it.

BEFORE BED

You'll be sick to death of fruit and vegetables by now and anyway they don't seem to be very good last thing at night. If you really feel you have to have something before retiring have an oatcake, or an organic rice cake thinly covered with sesame seed spread. As a bed-time drink you can try Barleycup. If you haven't had too many cups of herbal tea throughout the day, have one now formulated for late at night. An 'early-morning' herb tea at this time may keep you awake.

NOTE When embarking on this diet you may find it difficult to get to sleep. This is partly because you are changing your eating habits radically and your body has not adjusted to them, and partly because you are feeling deprived of tea and coffee. A bedtime herb drink will help you get over insomnia which in any case should not last for too long.

WHAT IF I'M STILL HUNGRY?

Those who find this diet impossible should cook a large quantity of brown rice and keep it in the fridge to turn to when, and if, hunger becomes acute and painful. Actually the problem does not lie so much with the actual hunger as with the fact that you are not now eating any of the comforting foods.

HOW LONG IS THE DIET FOR?

If you are serious about banishing cellulite forever you must stay on the diet for the rest of your life. Of course, the rigorous initial regime does not have to be kept up – nor should it as it does not constitute a long-term balanced diet – but it is important to develop a diet for life that will maintain the body in a detoxified and toned-up condition.

It is only the first two weeks of the cleansing and detoxifying diet that are very strict but after that you can start introducing a wider variety of foods to your diet (see Step 5).

If you have the occasional lapse during the first two weeks' anti-cellulite diet, at least make sure that you have a big salad at every meal. To some extent this will neutralize the bad effect of anything else you might have eaten.

AM I STILL ALLOWED TO EAT 'NAUGHTY' FOODS?

Many people who have been on the cleansing and detoxifying diet for any length of time find that they experience new taste sensations and they simply can't go back to their old ways. Cakes, white pastry, thick cream and biscuits start to taste heavy and cloying. You can almost sense the cellulite going back on if you bite into one of these products.

Don't imagine, though, you have to say goodbye to these foods for ever. The occasional slice of Black Forest gateau or dish swimming in cream sauce does you no harm at all, and if you find it absolutely delicious it probably does you good psychologically, too.

TO SUM UP

You should avoid, at least for the first fortnight of anti-cellulite eating: milk and dairy products, meat and fish if possible, all processed foods, anything cooked, salted nuts and crisps, all preserved meats, spirits, smoked foods, instant coffee (best to avoid this at all times) and ready-frozen meals. All these substances are cellulite-forming and will undo all the good work you are doing in other areas.

Also best avoided are all products made with white or refined flour, bread, biscuits, ice-cream, pastry, bought sauces, pasta and all fried foods.

If you can manage the diet for two weeks then you will be well on the way towards shifting that awful cellulite. And, as a plus, your general health will improve by leaps and bounds as well.

STEP 5
THE ANTI-CELLULITE KITCHEN
Cook your way to success

The question everybody contemplating the anti-cellulite diet asks is: how long will it take to achieve results?

It would be wonderful if we could diet for one, or at the most two, days and then all the cellulite would be gone forever. Unfortunately, it does not happen like that. For most people cellulite deposits have built up gradually over the years and, having lodged themselves firmly in position, are most reluctant to disappear. This is why after the two week cleansing and detoxifying diet, a dedicated and prolonged attack is necessary, and why you have to establish a way of eating that will mean your cellulite does not stand a chance of coming back.

The basic idea behind the anti-cellulite diet is that it is high in nutritional value and low in all substances that can cause physical degeneration, addictions, cravings and toxic conditions within the body. So it is an extremely healthy diet. You will feel much better on this diet than on the standard modern intake of processed and overcooked foods.

The following recipes will help you combat those ugly lumps and bumps forever. They are all quick and easy to cook as well as appetizing and enjoyable to eat.

YOUR STORE CUPBOARD

When establishing an anti-cellulite kitchen, the emphasis is on natural, additive-free, non-artificially coloured ingredients. Wherever possible, buy the real thing. For instance, buy **real coffee**, never instant coffee. Keep coffee beans in the freezer and grind them as you require them. It is now possible to buy decaffeinated beans and also ready-ground decaffeinated filter coffee.

Get into the habit of buying **herbal teas**. There is now a huge variety available so these drinks need never become boring.

All **fruit and vegetable juices** are good for you so long as they do not contain added sugar. Always have a big bowl of fresh fruit and lots of fresh vegetables, preferably organically grown. All **sprouted grains** – alfalfa, mung, beansprouts etc – are good, but they go off very quickly indeed and should really be eaten the same day they are bought.

Buy **soya** or **oat flour** instead of wheat flour and try **carob powder** instead of chocolate. Carob is rather like chocolate in taste but is much lower in fat and sugar and is not addictive.

Your store cupboard should always contain **seeds** and **unsalted nuts**. Choose from sesame, pumpkin, poppy, caraway and sunflower seeds, pine kernels, almonds, brazils, cashews, chestnuts, walnuts, hazelnuts and pecans. Always buy fresh rather than salted nuts. Peanuts are not recommended on the anti-cellulite diet as they are acid-forming and heavy on the liver.

Keep on the look-out for **gluten-free bread** and similar products. Rye bread, oatcakes, pumpernickel, barley cakes and puffed rice cakes are all good substitutes for bread.

Always buy brown rice rather than white and **buckwheat spaghetti** rather than the ordinary kind. Barley can be used in all brown rice recipes for a change.

Do stock up on **pulses**. Lentils – red, green and brown – do not need soaking so they are worth buying in packets, but if you prefer you can buy tins of the other pulses – butter beans, chick peas, kidney beans etc – to save time. Generally I do not recommend tinned foods, but pulses other than lentils take ages to cook and seem to lose very little in the tinning process. Tins of chick peas and kidney beans are cheap and ready to use, and can be rinsed and added to any salad dish to make a satisfying meal.

Dairy products should be avoided as much as possible. Instead, get into the habit of buying **soya milk** and **tofu** – an unfermented soya-bean curd.

Don't forget **Quorn**, now available in pieces, mince and ready-made recipes. Quorn is low-fat mycoprotein, more versatile than meat, and can be used in all meat recipes.

The only yoghurt you should buy from now on is **low-fat live plain yoghurt**. This is very low in calories and also quite thick. Don't buy any cream – double, single, clotted or sour. Cow's milk should be skimmed or semi-skimmed. **Plain cottage cheese**, **fromage frais**, **quark** – a tasty soft cheese prepared with skimmed milk – and **medium-fat vegetable rennet feta** are the only acceptable cheeses from now on. **Soya cheese**, available from health food shops, is quite delicious and okay to use occasionally.

Butter is better than margarine simply because it's more natural and not highly processed. Always buy the unsalted kind, and use extremely sparingly. Do not use in cooking. Always use **cold-pressed vegetable oils**. Use extra-virgin cold-pressed olive oil, sesame seed, grape seed, sunflower or safflower oil.

There are no recipes in this book for eggs. I have not eaten eggs for ten years and have not missed them once. They are not necessary to your diet at all. But if you like them, it goes without saying that you should only buy free-range eggs from hens that have been fed on organic produce.

Buy only **meat, fish or poultry from an organic source**. You do not need meat or fish, but if you like it, or feel you cannot do without it, then eat it from time to time. Smoked meats, fish and cheese are OUT because the smoking process results in free radicals.

Seasonings are of course extremely important in the anti-cellulite diet. Always buy sea salt and whole peppercorns. Keep a large supply of vegetable stock cubes or buy Vecon or Vegemite in jars. Fresh ginger root is used a lot in the recipes, as is garlic. I have discovered onion powder, available from many supermarkets, for dips and patés, and it is wonderful. It does not contain any additives, and it saves having to be in floods of tears from chopping up onions all the time.

All the **curry spices** – turmeric, cumin, coriander, fenugreek, garam masala – are useful, especially when you are cooking low-salt recipes. Cinnamon, allspice, bay leaves, cloves, cayenne, dill, fennel, nutmeg, oregano, paprika and mustard seeds are all vital. Whenever possible, buy herbs such as basil, parsley, coriander, rosemary, sage and thyme fresh.

All **flavourings**, such as vanilla essence, should be the real thing and not artificial substitutes.

Low-salt soya sauce is very handy as a flavouring. You can now also buy 'healthy' versions of tomato ketchup and Worcestershire sauce from health food shops.

Spreads and jams should not contain added sugar. I have grown to love sesame seed spread – tahini – and sunflower spread, which I now buy in preference to butter.

WHY A VEGETARIAN DIET IS BETTER

The best anti-cellulite diet is a strictly vegetarian one, where no animal products, including dairy products are eaten at all. But apart from their general 'healthiness', vegetarian meals have several advantages over meat dishes. They are often quicker and easier to prepare and the ingredients are nicer to handle. They tend to be cheaper but most important, *people often enjoy them more!*

Vegetarian meals taste cleaner and lighter than meat ones and are easier to digest. They don't leave a heavy feeling in the stomach and many people find they have far more energy on a vegetarian diet.

However, for some people a sudden change to total vegetarianism is neither possible nor desirable. So I have included some anti-cellulite meat and fish dishes at the end of this section.

2 GOLDEN RULES FOR ANTI-CELLULITE COOKING

Firstly, no high-fat dairy products are allowed. This means no eggs, double cream, full-cream milk, butter or full-fat cheese. The only permissible dairy foods are low-fat yoghurt and quark, which can be eaten occasionally. The reason for avoiding dairy products is that they are mucus-forming, which means they encourage cells and arteries to become clogged and blocked. Dairy products discourage quick through-put and elimination of food. Another factor is that these days many dairy foods are produced intensively, with the addition of hormones and chemicals, and these encourage the formation of cellulite.

Secondly: don't, as far as possible, fry in oil or butter. This is in order to avoid the formation of free radicals.

It is a culinary cliché that vegetables need to be sautéed first. However, this is done out of habit rather than necessity. 'Stir-fry' in water or stock instead – it will taste just as good, if not better.

Note: **The quantities given in these recipes are for four people. But as this kind of cookery is not an exact science the quantities do not need to be followed exactly, especially with the vegetables. Spices are mainly a matter of taste, but err on the mean side at first, especially if the most exotic**

> ingredients are new to you. In any case, anti-cellulite food
> should not be too highly spiced.

THE RECIPES

Breakfast

There is plenty of scope for the anti-cellulite breakfast to be both varied and delicious – and filling and satisfying at the same time.

This is the time of the day when you can eat a lot of **fruit**. It is in fact a good idea to eat most of your fruit in the morning because the later in the day you eat it, the harder your body finds it to digest. See page 27 for good fruits to eat.

If you are starting the anti-cellulite regime, it is best to stick to one variety of fruit at a time rather than having a fruit cocktail which can be hard work for the digestive system as all the fruits contain different substances.

Porridge is a very good, healthy food for all the family, provided it is made the traditional way, and not with lashings of milk, cream and sugar. You can add a small amount of organic honey, chopped dates or figs or soaked Hunza apricots to the basic oatmeal mixture. To make porridge, use twice the amount of water to porridge oats, bring to the boil then simmer, stirring all the time until you have a smooth paste.

Muesli is also a good choice for breakfast so long as it does not contain sugar or any preservatives or additives. Many ready-made mueslis are very high in both fats and sugar, so read the label carefully first. Soak overnight in a little mineral water and then eat with live low-fat yoghurt in the morning.

You do not necessarily have to give up **bread** at the start of the day. Oatcakes, pumpernickel, rye and Manana bread are all acceptable gluten-free substitutes or you can buy special gluten-free bread. Wholemeal pitta bread, which is unleavened, can be heated in the oven or microwave and then filled with sesame or sunflower spread.

Whatever you do, never go without breakfast. Breakfast need only take a very few minutes to prepare and eat and it will set you up for hours.

Soups

These soups are quick and easy to make. Unlike most recipes for soups, they do not rely on initial sautéeing in oil or butter. You may notice that they taste slightly different from the homemade soups you are used to, and the difference will be that they are lighter and fresher in taste.

The fresher the vegetables, the tastier the soups will be. These ones require little or no culinary skill.

LEEK AND POTATO SOUP

A quick, easy and satisfying soup for when leeks are in season.

1 medium onion, finely chopped
2 large leeks, washed and chopped
2 large potatoes, scrubbed and cubed
2oz (50g) ground cashews or hazelnuts
1 pint (600ml) vegetable stock
pinch mixed dried herbs
sea salt and freshly ground black pepper

preparation time:10 minutes
cooking time: 35 minutes

Heat 2-3 tablespoons of the stock in a large saucepan. Add the onion, leeks, potatoes and nuts and stir-fry in the stock over a medium heat for 5 minutes. Bring to the boil and add the rest of the stock. Cover and simmer until the potatoes are cooked but still intact (about 25 minutes). Allow to cool slightly, then liquidize. Return to the saucepan and reheat gently with the herbs and seasoning. Do not boil.

SPINACH AND TOFU SOUP

A light and creamy soup which requires minimal cooking time.

2¹/₄ pints (1.35l) vegetable stock
2 packs Tofeata or Morinaga tofu, drained and cut into cubes
2lb (900g) spinach, washed and roughly chopped
sea salt and freshly ground black pepper
chopped fresh parsley to garnish

preparation time: 5 minutes
cooking time: 20 minutes

Bring the stock to the boil in a pan. Add the tofu and spinach and bring back to the boil, then cover and simmer for 10 minutes, stirring occasionally. Liquidize if liked, when cooled slightly. Add salt and pepper and reheat. Sprinkle the chopped parsley over the soup just before serving.

Starters and Dips

These delicious starters and dips are all anti-cellulite but they are not necessarily low-calorie.

When recipes specify olive oil make sure you always use one labelled 'extra-virgin'. Although olive oil is the best sort of oil to use, as it is monounsaturated, it does have rather a strong taste and if you don't like it you can substitute a cold-pressed sesame or grape seed oil, which have hardly any taste at all.

AVOCADO DIP

Avocados are high in fat, but they do not encourage cellulite to form. This dip is good with crudités, or it can be spread on manna bread or oatcakes, like the hummous.

1 large ripe avocado peeled, stoned and chopped
1 pack tofu broken into pieces
juice of 1 lemon, or to taste
2 tablespoons cold-pressed sunflower or grape seed oil
sea salt and freshly ground black pepper

preparation time: about 5 minutes
cooking time: nil

Put all the ingredients in a blender and blend until smooth.

HUMMOUS

There are many versions of hummous, a Greek dish based on chick peas.
Over the years I must have tried them all, and this one is my favourite.

1 14oz (400g) tin chick peas, drained and rinsed

1 dessertspoon tahini

juice 1 lemon

1 clove garlic, crushed

2 tablespoons olive oil

1 tablespoon low-fat natural yoghurt

1 dessertspoon chopped fresh parsley

sea salt and freshly ground black pepper

paprika to garnish

preparation time: about 5 minutes

cooking time: nil

This must be one of the easiest dishes ever devised if you have a liquidizer.
If not, I should imagine it's murder. Simply put all the ingredients except
the paprika into the liquidizer and blend on top speed until a smooth
paste is formed. Turn into a suitable dish and garnish with paprika.

Serve with crudités – sticks of carrot and celery, chunks of broccoli or
cauliflower, and green and red peppers. You can also serve hummous
with manna or gluten-free bread, or spread on oatcakes or barley cakes.
You will not need to spread butter or margarine on first.

CASHEW AND TOFU PÂTÉ

This is a more 'festive', sophisticated pâté, for special occasions or dinner parties.

2 tablespoons vegetable stock
1 small onion or shallot, very finely chopped
1 clove garlic, crushed
1 pack Morinaga or Tofeata tofu
4oz (125g) ground cashew nuts
1 tablespoon olive oil
4 tablespoons spring or filtered water (or, for a very special occasion, you could use white wine)
2 tablespoons chopped fresh parsley, or (in an emergency) 2 teaspoons dried sea salt and freshly ground black pepper

preparation time: about 10 minutes
cooking time: 5 minutes

Heat the vegetable stock in a saucepan and gently stir-fry the onion and garlic over a medium heat until softened. Remove from the heat. In a large mixing bowl, mash the tofu with a fork, then add the onion and garlic. Now add the nuts, olive oil, water or wine, parsley, salt and pepper and stir well. Press the pâté into 1 large or 4 small earthenware dishes and chill in the fridge for an hour or two, if possible, before serving.

Salads

Salads are, of course, the mainstay of the anti-cellulite diet. Even if you haven't always got the time or the ingredients for a full-scale salad, you should make sure you have something raw at every meal, as to some extent this will work to detoxify any less healthy food you might have eaten or be about to eat.

When possible, make sure the salad ingredients are really fresh and organically grown. And do get into the habit of buying fresh sprouted grains, such as beansprouts, alfalfa or others, which contain many important nutrients. Sprouted grains can be strewn over the top of just about any salad.

GREEK SALAD

You can now buy low-fat vegetarian feta cheese, which makes this popular Greek salad suitable for cellulite-shifters.

1 pack vegetarian feta cheese
½ iceberg lettuce, washed and sliced or torn into strips
½ cucumber, cut into chunks
4–5 firm tomatoes, cut into chunks
12 black olives
vinaigrette dressing (see page 55)

In a bowl, combine all the salad ingredients and toss in the vinaigrette.

MIXED SALAD

Green salads can consist of just lettuce, cucumber and green peppers. This salad is slightly more special.

½ iceberg lettuce, washed and sliced or torn into strips
1 bunch watercress, washed and chopped
2-3 spring onions, finely chopped
2 courgettes, grated
2 carrots, grated
4 tomatoes, sliced
sunflower or pumpkin seeds
vinaigrette dressing (see page 55)

Combine all the salad ingredients and toss in the vinaigrette dressing. Experiment with other green leaves in salads – the choice has never been wider. Choose from lamb's lettuce, cos lettuce, Chinese leaves, radicchio, chicory, spinach leaves (use raw), nasturtium leaves, celery leaves, dandelion leaves (as long as they are young and very green). It is a good idea to keep a wooden bowl specially for green salads. Rub a clove of garlic round the inside first, and then just wipe after using. It should not need washing up.

Other vegetables can easily be added to a green salad – raw cauliflower or broccoli florets, or avocado slices, for example. Nuts, such as walnuts or hazelnuts, can also be added.

SPINACH AND CAULIFLOWER SALAD

This salad uses raw cauliflower, so make sure all the florets are very crisp and crunchy, and don't leave in any woody cauliflower stems.

8oz (225g) new potatoes, cooked with mint, then cooled
1 medium cauliflower, cut into very small florets
1lb (450g) spinach, washed and torn into strips
2–3 dessert apples, cored and sliced
2oz (50g) sunflower or soya cheese, cubed or sliced
vinaigrette dressing (see page 55)

If the potatoes are very tiny, leave whole. Otherwise, slice them and mix with the remaining salad ingredients. Toss in the vinaigrette.

VINAIGRETTE DRESSING

It is a good idea to make up this dressing in advance and then keep it in a screw top jar in the fridge until required. It keeps well, and is suitable for most salads.

6 fl oz (175ml) cold-pressed olive oil, or other
cold-pressed oil
3 fl oz (75ml) white wine vinegar
½ teaspoon honey
½ teaspoon sea salt
½ teaspoon freshly ground black pepper
1 teaspoon fresh or ½ teaspoon dried tarragon
½ teaspoon made mustard

Put all the ingredients in a bottle with a screw top lid and shake thoroughly. This dressing is best left a day or two before use for the flavours to meld together. Before using, shake thoroughly again.

Vegetarian Main Courses

JACKET POTATOES

These are the easiest vegetables to start you off on an anti-cellulite cookery regime. Try to buy organically grown potatoes if possible.

Cooking potatoes in their jackets conserves all their goodness – especially as most of the nutrients are found in or near the skin – and it is simplicity itself. Just preheat the oven to 400°F, 200°C, or gas mark 6, scrub the potatoes, prick with a fork and cook at the top of the oven for about an hour. Do not rub with butter or cover in aluminium foil (which is now being associated with the degeneration of tissues). If you use a microwave, jacket potatoes will take about 10 minutes to cook, according to size.

Cellulite-shifters should eat their potatoes with a salad, or they can be used to accompany any dish at all.

You should never eat chips or mash your potatoes with cream, milk or butter. You can mash them with a little low-fat yoghurt if you like, but that's all.

BROCCOLI, SESAME SEED AND BROWN RICE CURRY

Curries are extremely easy to prepare and have the advantage of making ordinary vegetables tastier and more special. This one is a quick and easy favourite.

Always use brown rice. It takes a little longer to cook than white, although many of the newer types of brown rice on sale are 'quick-cook', but the difference in taste is worth it.

½ pint (300ml) vegetable stock, made with Vecon or vegetable stock cube
1lb (450g) broccoli, chopped
8oz (225g) mushrooms, washed and chopped
2 tablespoons sesame seeds
sea salt and freshly ground black pepper
1 level teaspoon mild curry powder or garam masala
8oz (225g) brown rice, cooked

preparation time: about 10 minutes
cooking time: about 20 minutes

Heat about ¼ pint (150ml) of the stock in a saucepan and add the broccoli. Stir-fry for 3 minutes, then add the chopped mushrooms and stir for another 2 minutes. Add the remaining stock, bring to the boil then cover and simmer until the broccoli is just tender – about 10 minutes.

Add the sesame seeds, salt and pepper and stir for 1 minute. Add the rice and curry powder and stir until thoroughly heated through. Serve at once with a mixed salad.

Note: the rice for this dish is even nicer if cooked in vegetable stock rather than plain water.

BRAISED VEGETABLES WITH CHINESE NOODLES

Chinese cooking lends itself very easily to the anti-cellulite regime so long as you always stir-fry in stock rather than in any kind of oil.

This is a highly sophisticated dish, suitable for dinner parties. It is especially suitable for anybody who is on a low-salt, low-fat or low-carbohydrate diet for any reason.

for the sauce:
2 tablespoons dry sherry

2 tablespoons soy sauce

1 tablespoon vegetable stock

1 teaspoon corn flour

**8oz (225g) noodles – if using the Chinese noodles in compressed
    squares, allow 1 square per person**

8 fl oz (250ml) vegetable stock

4oz (125g) mange tout peas, stems and strings removed

8oz (225g) Chinese or white cabbage, shredded

8oz (225g) mushrooms, finely chopped

2 medium carrots, finely chopped

2 shallots or small onions, finely chopped

1 small green pepper, seeded and sliced

1 small red pepper, seeded and sliced

4oz (125g) bean sprouts

1 tablespoon sesame seeds, roasted. (You can dry-roast sesame seeds by stirring them for 1-2 minutes in a pan on a high heat. Keep stirring, or they will stick and burn.)

preparation time: 15 minutes

cooking time: 10 minutes

First, make the sauce by mixing together all the ingredients in a bowl. Set aside. Cook the noodles according to the instructions on the packet. Heat the stock in a large non-stick pan. When it is bubbling gently, add the mange tout, cabbage, mushrooms, carrots, shallots and peppers and stir-fry on a high heat for 3 minutes. Add the bean sprouts and stir-fry for 1 minute, then add the sauce, lower the heat and simmer for 2 minutes. Add the roasted sesame seeds and serve immediately with the noodles.

TOFU SHEPHERD'S PIE

A totally tasteless cheese-like white block in its natural state, tofu is a cellulite-shifter's delight. It is low in calories, dairy-free, highly nutritious and blends in well with many kinds of food.

This recipe is such an improvement on the traditional version, and it is popular with all age groups and even fussy eaters.

½ cup vegetable stock

1 onion, finely chopped

8oz (225g) mushrooms, chopped

1 green pepper, seeded and sliced

2 large carrots, finely chopped

6 tomatoes, skinned, or 14oz (400g) tin tomatoes, chopped

1 bay leaf

2 heaped teaspoons fresh chopped basil, or ½ teaspoon dried

1 pack Morinaga or Tofeata tofu

sea salt and freshly ground black pepper to taste

1lb (450g) mashed potatoes (do not mash them with butter, cream or milk)

preparation time: about 15 minutes

cooking time: 45 minutes

Preheat the oven to 375°F, 190°C, gas mark 5. Heat the stock in a non-stick pan, add the onion and stir-fry for 2 minutes. Add the mushrooms, green pepper and carrots and continue to stir-fry over a medium heat for about 3 minutes, then add the tomatoes, bay leaf and basil. Cover and simmer for about 15 minutes.

Chop or break up the tofu and add to the vegetable mixture, stirring all the time. Add the sea salt and black pepper, then turn the mixture into a large casserole and top with the mashed potatoes. Bake in the oven for 20 minutes or until the potatoes are lightly browned.

Serve with a green salad; it doesn't need anything else.

KIDNEY BEAN CASSEROLE

Pulses – lentils, black-eyed beans, haricot beans, kidney beans, even baked beans if they are sugar-free – are marvellous foods for those wishing to be rid of cellulite. They provide complex carbohydrates and are nutritionally satisfying, tasty and versatile.

This is a very warming and filling winter dish. As it contains chillies, it is also quite hot. If you are cooking this dish for children or people who don't like very spicy food, omit the chillies and instead use 1 dessertspoon paprika.

Note: Always rinse tinned pulses in filtered water before using as they tend to be preserved in brine.

14oz (400g) tin red kidney beans, drained and rinsed
1 pint (600ml) water, if using dried beans
1lb (450g) tomatoes, skinned and sliced
sea salt and freshly ground black pepper
2 large red peppers, seeded and sliced
2 medium onions, sliced
1 clove garlic, crushed
2 fresh red chillies, seeded and finely chopped, or 2 dried red chillies
2 teaspoons paprika

preparation time: about 15 minutes
cooking time: 1½ hours

Preheat the oven to 325°F, 160°C, gas mark 3.

Layer half the tomatoes in a large casserole, season well, then add a layer of peppers, onions and garlic, chillies and paprika. Put in all the beans, followed by a second layer of peppers, onions and garlic, with the remaining tomatoes on top. Season again. Cover the casserole and bake in the oven for about 1½ hours. Serve with brown rice and a green salad.

SIMPLE BRAZIL NUT ROAST

Nut loaves are the vegetarian equivalent of roasts. They are quite time-consuming to prepare and cook, but good for special occasions. All nut loaves can be made in advance and then frozen until needed.

This is one of the easiest to make. As with all nut loaves, it is very filling. You can use other nuts, such as hazels or cashews, in this basic recipe.

1 large onion, finely chopped
4oz (125g) carrots, grated
about 3 tablespoons vegetable stock
4oz (125g) brazil nuts, finely milled
4oz (125g) wholemeal breadcrumbs
1 teaspoon chopped fresh sage or rosemary or ½ teaspoon dried sea
salt and freshly ground black pepper
3 level tablespoons soya flour
1 tablespoon sesame seeds

preparation time: 15 minutes
cooking time: about 45 minutes

Preheat the oven to 350°F, 180°C, gas mark 4.

Sweat the onion and carrots over a medium heat in 2–3 tablespoons vegetable stock for 5 minutes. Add the nuts, breadcrumbs, herbs, seasonings and flour. If the mixture is too dry, add a little more vegetable stock. It should be sticky but not runny. Press into a 1lb (450g) loaf tin and sprinkle with the sesame seeds. Bake in the oven for 30–40 minutes. Serve with salad.

Meat and Fish Main Courses

This section has been contributed by aromatherapist Frances Clifford, who helped me to get rid of my cellulite.

Meat and fish, says Frances, have very little place in any successful cellulite-shedding regime. The reason is that both these foods clog up the system and putrefy quickly once in the bowel. Also, they do not combine successfully with carbohydrates in the digestive system. Therefore they should be eaten only infrequently – once a week for chicken or other meat, say Sunday lunch, and twice a week for fish. Do not eat animal protein more often than this while you are trying to lose cellulite.

When buying meat, make sure it is locally reared, fresh and unprocessed. Do not buy meats that have been extensively processed, smoked, or contain preservatives or additives.

Fish should also be bought as close to its source as possible. Fresh fish is bright-eyed, bright-skinned and not slimy-looking or strange-smelling. Before buying, check that the fish is freshly caught.

When cooking meat or fish the anti-cellulite way, do not fry or barbecue as very hot cooking oil releases free radicals. It is better to 'dry-roast' meat – that is, put it in a covered pot or casserole with seasonings, and cook on a very low heat (275°F, 140°C, gas mark 1) for several hours. If you have a crock pot, you will find this invaluable, but whatever you do, never fry the meat in oil first.

LEMON-BAKED PLAICE

1–2 fillets plaice per person

grated rind ½ lemon and 2 teaspoons lemon juice per fillet

sea salt and freshly ground black pepper

2 dessertspoons mixed fresh herbs – thyme, marjoram, parsley,

oregano, for example – or ½ teaspoon mixed dried herbs per fillet

lemon wedges and parsley sprigs to garnish

preparation time: 10 minutes

cooking time: 40–50 minutes

Preheat the oven to 325°F, 170°C, gas mark 3. Season each fillet with lemon rind, salt and pepper. Roll each one up and secure with a cocktail stick or skewer. Pack the prepared fillets into a casserole, sprinkle over the mixed herbs, cover with the remaining lemon juice and rind, and cover with a lid.

Cook for about 40–50 minutes, or until the plaice is completely white and flakes easily. When ready, lift out with a fish slice onto a warmed serving dish. Garnish with the lemon wedges and parsley. Serve with a mixed green salad, steamed mange tout and new baby carrots or baby corn.

Note: This recipe can be adapted to any kind of flat fish.

DINNER PARTY SALMON

1 bay leaf per steak

1 salmon steak per person. Buy wild salmon if possible

about ½ teaspoon extra-virgin olive oil per steak

sea salt and freshly ground black pepper

juice ½ lemon or 1 teaspoon dry martini per steak

1 dessertspoon chopped chives or parsley per salmon steak

preparation time: 10 minutes

cooking time: about 20 minutes

Lightly oil a large grill pan with olive oil. Arrange the bay leaves in the pan and place 1 salmon steak on each. Brush the steaks with the olive oil and season with salt and pepper. Cook gently under the grill, without charring, to allow natural oils to be released.

After about 20 minutes, or when the fish is flaky, pour over the lemon juice or dry martini and replace for a maximum of 1 minute under the grill. Put the steaks on a hot serving plate with the cooking juices, and garnish with chopped chives or parsley. Serve with tossed green salad and mixed steamed vegetables.

Can be kept warm in a very low oven for 30 minutes, if well covered.

Note: this recipe can be used for any fish steaks.

Organically reared, free-range chicken smells quite delicious when cooking and produces relatively few juices compared to mass-produced birds that have been plumped up with water and preservatives.

1 organically reared chicken, corn-fed if possible

2-4 garlic cloves, peeled and halved

2 lemon halves, or 1 onion, peeled, with up to 10 cloves pressed into it

extra-virgin olive oil

sea salt and freshly ground black pepper

1 teaspoon dried or 1 dessertspoon fresh tarragon or rosemary

lemon wedges, fresh herbs, raw onion rings to garnish

preparation time: 15–20 minutes

cooking time: 1½–1¾ hours

Preheat the oven to 400°F, 200°C, gas mark 6.

Prepare the chicken by rinsing in cold water inside and out, then dry with a piece of kitchen towel roll. Discard the giblets. Using a sharp pointed knife, make 4–8 deep slits in the fleshiest part of the chicken – thigh or breast – and push the garlic halves well down into these.

Put the lemon halves or the onion inside the chicken. Smear the upper part of the chicken with olive oil and put into a casserole. Season with salt and pepper and tarragon or rosemary. Cover with a lid and cook for 30-45 minutes, then reduce the heat to 300°F, 150°C, gas mark 2 and cook for 1 further hour. Test by sticking a knife in the thigh. If the juices run clear, the chicken is cooked.

To serve, place the chicken on a preheated dish. Remove the lemon or onion and pour the cooking juices over and around the bird. Garnish with lemon wedges and fresh tarragon or a few raw onion rings and sprigs of rosemary.

Serve with steamed carrots and broccoli, and a green salad.

LAMB

This is the only other 'everyday' meat that Frances recommends to her patients and even this should be eaten very seldom (about once or twice a month maximum) as it is high in fat and can be indigestible if you are trying to refine your diet. English lamb in season – Easter and early summer – is best because it has been subjected to less handling than imported lamb.

Lamb should be cooked using the 'pot roast' method as with chicken, and can be flavoured with lemon or rosemary. Garlic can be inserted into the meat if desired, and the joint can be seasoned with sea salt and freshly ground pepper.

Game eaten in season is very good and makes a welcome change from other forms of flesh protein. Always try to ensure that the game is wild and has been shot on the wing. Wild birds are lean and should be cooked slowly to preserve moisture. Duck, guinea fowl, pheasant and quail are all good and may be grilled or spit-roasted. Brush first with a very small amount of olive oil.

Pigeon are best braised on a bed of mixed vegetables, such as leeks and carrots, with a little red wine. Juniper berries are the best seasoning for game birds. Consult standard cookery books for game bird ideas but always use the pot roast method of cooking. Never fry or barbecue.

Puddings

Many people imagine that anyone who is serious about shifting cellulite will have to forego puddings for ever. However, this is not quite true. Although double cream and huge slices of Black Forest gâteau are out – except for the very occasional indulgence – there are ways in which you can end a meal with something satisfyingly sweet. For many of us, life would be bleak indeed without any puddings.

Here are some desserts that will cheer you up and satisfy the longing for something sweet at the end of a meal without encouraging the dreaded cellulite to return.

TOFU CHEESECAKE

Yes, you can have cheesecake – so long as you make it like this. As it takes a long time to chill, it is best to make it in the morning or even the night before you need it.

½ **cup rolled oats**

½oz **(15g) desiccated coconut**

½oz **(15g) butter**

1 **pack tofu**

2 **tablespoons low-fat natural yoghurt**

2 **tablespoons raw sugar or organic honey**

juice and rind ½ **orange**

½ **teaspoon natural vanilla essence**

2 **teaspoons tahini**

pinch sea salt

2–3 **tablespoons organic honey**

4 **tablespoons water**

½ **teaspoon powdered agar-agar (vegetarian gelling agent, available from health food shops)**

4oz **(125g) fresh or frozen raspberries**

preparation time: 15 minutes

cooking time: about 40 minutes

Preheat the oven to 350°F, 180°C, gas mark 4.

Mix the oats and coconut together in a bowl. Spread the butter over the bottom of an 8 inch (20cm) flan tin, then sprinkle the oat and coconut mixture over this. Press down and set aside. In a liquidizer, combine the tofu, yoghurt, sugar or honey, orange juice and rind, vanilla essence, tahini and salt. When thoroughly blended, pour into the flan case. In a small pan melt the honey in the water over a medium heat and stir in the agar-agar. Bring to the boil and simmer for about 1 minute. Remove from the heat, stir in the raspberries, and pour over the tofu mixture in the flan case. Bake in the oven for 35 minutes. Leave to cool, then chill for several hours before serving.

FRUIT PURÉE WITH MUESLI TOPPING

This can be served with low-fat yoghurt. Use the tiny Hunza dried apricots. They look unappetizing when dried but are far tastier than the bright-orange, sulphured variety.

4oz (125g) dried Hunza apricots, soaked overnight
4oz (125g) sunflower seeds, ground
1 banana
1 apple
juice ½ lemon
½ teaspoon organic honey

for the topping
4oz (125g) muesli base
2oz (50g) raisins
2oz (50g) flaked almonds
2oz (50g) sunflower seeds
2oz (50g) desiccated coconut (Or you could use Sunwheel 45 per cent fruit and nut deluxe muesli instead.)

preparation time: 10 minutes
cooking time: 5 minutes

Blend together in a liquidizer the apricots, sunflower seeds, banana, apple, lemon juice and honey, adding a little water if the mixture seems too stiff.

Toast the ingredients for the muesli topping under the grill until slightly browned. This will make it crunchy. Spread the topping over the purée and serve.

NO-COOK CAKE

This uncooked cake tastes just as good as, if not better than, standard baked cakes.

8oz (225g) oatflakes, fine, coarse or medium – it doesn't matter
4oz (125g) cashews, brazils or almonds, ground
1 banana, mashed
1 carrot, grated
juice 1 lemon
1 dessertspoon organic honey
water or soya milk to mix
strawberries, raspberries or fresh apricots to garnish

preparation time: 15 minutes
cooking time: nil

In a large mixing bowl, combine all the ingredients except the fruit for garnish, adding just enough water or soya milk – or you could use ordinary skimmed milk – to make the mixture moist and sticky. Press into a shallow cake tin, decorate with fresh fruit and chill for 1-2 hours. Serve with yoghurt.

STEP 6
DRY SKIN BRUSHING
Take direct action

Dry skin brushing is an extremely important step in the war against cellulite and you should begin doing it – in conjunction with aromatherapy and massage – as soon as you start the anti-cellulite diet.

Dry skin brushing is probably an ancient technique but it was revived in America in the early 1980s when colon-cleansing became all the rage. According to Dr Robert Gray, author of *The Colon Health Handbook,* skin brushing is a very effective way of enabling the lymphatic system to expel waste material which has been held for a long time inside the body.

Of course Dr Gray was only talking about the power of skin brushing to help the colon clear and it was several years before skin brushing was advocated for cellulite removal. Nowadays, skin brushing has become a standard technique recommended by doctors, nutritionists and healers who are interested in natural healing rather than relying on drugs, surgery and hospitals. Enthusiasts claim that the technique has many benefits apart from its ability to remove cellulite or clean out colons. Skin brushing can tone up your whole system, encourage ordinary fat to disperse, invigorate the brain and also remove stress and tension from the system.

HOW DOES IT WORK?

According to Dr Jack Soltanoff, author of *Natural Healing*, the technique is a mild form of acupressure and acupuncture performed without piercing the skin. The only tool that you need is a scrub or hand brush. Dry skin brushing, Dr Soltanoff says, has far-reaching beneficial effects on your health because it affects all your inner organs in the remote parts of your body via reflexes of the nervous system.

The eliminative organs, such as the bowels, lungs and kidneys are abused daily by most of us with the over-consumption of refined, commercialized processed foods, tobaccos, alcohol, coffee, tea and chocolate. The skin-brushing technique has the power, he says, to stimulate these organs into eliminating effectively.

On the ability of skin brushing to disperse cellulite, Dr Soltanoff writes:

> This technique works on the cellulite by gradually breaking down the obese liquid-filled fatty tissues and slowly releasing the toxic fluids through various channels, particularly the lymphatic system. With regular daily use, your legs will firm up and tighten. You'll have a much younger figure and that in itself will make you feel terrific.

WHAT KIND OF BRUSH DO YOU NEED?

It is essential to have the correct type of brush. This must be very hard and made of natural, not synthetic fibres. A soft bristle brush won't have the same effect at all. Most body brushing experts recommend a long-handled brush of Mexican cactus fibre. The handle should be detachable and made of natural wood with a strap across the brush.

TIP: These brushes are stiff and scratchy when you first use them and you may feel that they will take your skin off. If yours scratches too much, soak it for a few hours in the bathroom basin, then dry overnight in the airing cupboard. It will then be soft enough to use without harming the skin.

HOW DO YOU DO IT?

In order for dry skin brushing to be really effective, the strokes you apply have to be firm and long. Start with light pressure and gradually build up as your skin becomes used to the sensation. You will discover in time that the skin can take quite hard pressure but it will probably be tender at first.

Dry skin brushing in this way is not the same thing as brushing your skin with a loofah, bath mitt or ordinary back brush. None of these will work to break down cellulite, or activate the lymphatic system because they go soft very quickly. It is only all-over brushing with the right kind of brush which will have this affect.

If you are interested only in brushing to get rid of cellulite, you can concentrate on these areas. The pressure can be as hard as you like. Brush up the **back of the leg** in long, single strokes. Then when you get to the **thigh**, brush upwards as vigorously as you can where the cellulite is at its most dense. Finish off by brushing the **buttocks** equally hard, in any direction. Usually, skin brushing has to be done in the direction of the heart, but circular movements round the buttocks are best.

Brush both legs an equal amount and then get into the bath. You will find the bath water makes your skin tingle pleasantly. If you are doing body brushing in conjunction with aromatherapy you should rub in the essential oils straight after you get out of the bath, again paying particular attention to the cellulite areas. The best time for applying the massage oils is after body brushing and a bath because the pores will be open and unclogged.

A WORD OF ADVICE: If you find the brushing has left long scratches, or makes you look as though you have walked through a field of brambles, you are either doing it too hard or the brush needs more soaking. The brushing should never be allowed to break the skin. In any case, never brush over broken skin.

THE WHOLE-BODY BRUSH

You don't, of course, have to limit skin brushing to cellulite-dense areas. A whole-body brush will tone up the system even more and increase the benefits.

This is how you do it.

You should start by brushing your **fingers and hands**. Hold your hands with fingers splayed and brush between each finger a few times. Brush on top of the hand and then the palm as many times as you like. Repeat this with the other hand.

Now do your **arms**. Brush in long strokes from the wrist to the elbow, then from the elbow to the shoulder. Always use long, firm, bold strokes and remember always to brush in the direction of the heart.

After this, do your **toes and feet**. Put one leg on the rim of the bath or basin and brush across the tops of the toes. Brush the soles of the feet, then around the ankles. Again, use the firmest possible strokes. Brush the **leg up to the knee**, going all round the leg and using long strokes from the ankle. Repeat this about 14 times. Now brush the **thighs** and **buttocks**. Repeat with the other leg. As you brush you will soon get to know the cellulite areas and you will see them gradually diminishing over the weeks. But don't expect that one vigorous brushing session will send them away. For really bad cellulite, you may have to keep this practice up for months.

After having a really good go at the worst areas of cellulite you should now move up to the **neck**. Brush downwards from the head, front and back. Now do the **shoulders**, this time brushing downwards to keep in the direction of the heart.

Cellulite sufferers can help to activate the lymphatic system by holding the brush in the **armpit** and rotating it seven times to the left and seven times to the right. This action, if repeated daily, gets the lymph nodes working again.

Now do the front and sides of the body. Women should avoid brushing over the nipples, but can brush over the **breasts**, perhaps with lighter pressure. Some authorities do not advise brushing over the stomach and abdomen, as the action can be too strong. It is probably better to leave this area alone and go on to the **back**. You will need the long handle to reach the back and again, long, firm strokes should be used.

WHEN AND FOR HOW LONG?

Although the above procedure may sound complicated, in fact it is very simple indeed and takes no more than five minutes per session. Women with very bad cellulite should spend at last five minutes a day on body brushing for two months. After this length of time, the body gets used to the brushing and the technique is less effective. When this happens you should brush every other day.

Once the worst of the cellulite has gone, keep it away by skin brushing once or twice a week. You don't want it to start creeping back after all your hard work.

WHAT IF MY SKIN STARTS DOING FUNNY THINGS?

You may find that your skin does funny things when you embark on brushing it. Remember that this is not just a beauty treatment but an

> **A WORD OF ADVICE:** Some women find that once they start on a serious anti-cellulite regime they can't stop and tend to over-do it at first. But the body has to be helped to get rid of its cellulite gently and safely and you have to be patient. Just because five minutes of body brushing is good, it doesn't follow that ten minutes or a quarter of an hour will be much better. Be gentle at first and build up pressure gradually once your skin has got used to the sensation.

actual health-promoting regime. Most people find that their skin changes texture after a few weeks of brushing. In my case it went extremely dry for a time and all the massage oils in the world didn't seem to make any difference. But after this, it seemed to go very smooth and unlined. Those who find that their skin seems to alter should just continue with the brushing. It can't do you any harm.

IMPORTANT: The technique is safe for everybody except for those who have damaged, infected or broken skin. People who have eczema, psoriasis or any other skin complaint should not use the brush on affected areas. You can brush where the skin is free from damage though the technique should not be used on any areas where you have bad varicose veins.

A FINAL WORD

Body brushing must be carried out in conjunction with the cleansing diet detailed in Steps 4 and 5. There is no point working hard to unclog the system from the outside if you are filling it up with rubbish on the inside.

STEP 7
AROMATHERAPY
Beat cellulite with essential oils

NOT JUST A 'FRENCH LOAD OF OLD COBBLERS'

Aromatherapy is one of the most successful forms of treatment for cellulite and most aromatherapists now offer anti-cellulite treatments. The essential oils used in aromatherapy work in conjunction with the diet and the body brushing to enable waste matter to empty itself into the lymphatic system.

Recent research on essential oils has established that many have a definite therapeutic effect and that they *do* make a difference. For many years aromatherapy was regarded as a 'French load of old cobblers' in much the same way as cellulite itself was (and still is in some circles), but it is rapidly becoming one of the most popular complementary therapies.

We now know that aromatherapy oils are not just nice scents but can be very potent remedies for a variety of ailments. There are specific oils for cleansing, detoxifying and stimulating circulation to help bring about the body changes, which will lead to a loss of cellulite.

THE ANTI-CELLULITE AROMATHERAPY OILS

with their botanical names

- **LEMON:** *Citrus limonum*
- **JUNIPER:** *Juniperus communis* **ssp.** *communis*
- **ROSEMARY:** *Rosmarinus officinalis* **CT cineole**
- **CLARY SAGE:** *Salvia sclarea*
- **CYPRESS:** *Cupressus sempervirens*
- **PATCHOULI:** *Pogostemon cablin*
- **GERANIUM:** *Pelargonium x asperum (roseum)*
- **BLACK PEPPER:** *Piper nigrum*
- **SANDALWOOD:** *Santalum album*

WHAT ARE ESSENTIAL OILS?

Basically they are the strong-smelling ingredients found in many plants. Most flowers, seeds, grains, roots and resins contain essential oils in minute quantities.

Some of these oils are healing and some are harmful. Harmful essential oils include wormwood, as used in absinthe. Healing oils include rosemary, geranium, patchouli, lavender and sweet almond. Oils from plants become 'essential' after they have been distilled and the highly concentrated 'essence' is obtained.

Once the oils have been distilled they are very volatile and will quickly evaporate. This is why you will always find aromatherapy oils in dark blue or brown bottles to keep the destructive effect of light away from their contents.

Chemically speaking, these oils are very complicated and this is where their therapeutic power lies. They are readily absorbed through the skin and taken up into the bloodstream.

Certain oils have a diuretic effect, some are relaxing, while others are stimulating and energizing. Just to give a few examples:

- **clary sage is a powerful relaxant and helps digestion**
- **geranium is an adrenal cortex stimulant and reliever of fluid retention**

- **lavender is calming and soothing**
- **cypress is a powerful astringent**
- **juniper purifies and stimulates the urino-genital tract**
- **rosemary encourages the lymphatic system to start working properly**

There are two ways of using aromatherapy to beat cellulite. You can either do it yourself or you can go to a qualified therapist.

WAGING WAR ON CELLULITE YOURSELF

It is perfectly possible to use essential oils by yourself to help the cellulite disappear.

There are now a number of special anti-cellulite oils on the market which are based on aromatherapy principles. These are not highly expensive 'miracle creams' but a mixture of essential oils diluted in the correct carrier oils. You can either buy anti-cellulite oils ready mixed, or make up your own from small bottles of essential oils.

Two of the main manufacturers of organic anti-cellulite oils in the UK are **Bodytreats International** and **Neal's Yard**.

Bodytreats have two types of anti-cellulite oils: a bath oil and a massage oil. The bath oil contains 'neat' essential oil for the bath and the massage oil is a dilution of the same oils in a vegetable carrier oil. You should put five drops (never more) into the bath.

Neal's Yard have a differently formulated anti-cellulite oil containing lemon, frankincense, juniper, black pepper and sandalwood in a base oil. Their leaflet states that the oil will help to 'eliminate toxins developing in the fatty tissues and in the body'.

PREPARING YOUR OWN ANTI-CELLULITE OILS

You should always match up bath oils to massage oils when embarking on anti-cellulite treatments. Essential oils which are good to use include lemon, rosemary, geranium, patchouli, cypress or juniper.

To use essential oils in the bath, simply shake in between six to ten drops of your chosen oil. For massage, the essential oils need to be mixed with a carrier oil.

Massage oils

These can easily be made by filling a 100 ml bottle – it should be opaque and dark – with the base or carrier oil, and then shaking about 30 drops of the essential oil into this.

The base, or carrier, oil that you use is important. It should be vegetable oil such as sweet almond, apricot kernel, avocado, grape seed, hazelnut or sunflower. Ordinary kitchen oil will do so long as it is not blended and it is cold-pressed. If it is cold-pressed, it will say so on the label. You can use olive oil if you like, although this is rather strong-smelling. But it works perfectly well as a carrier oil.

IMPORTANT: You should never use the same oil for more than two weeks at a time as they lose their potency once the body gets used to them. For rapid effect, change your oils frequently. For instance, if you use cypress for the first three weeks, change to rosemary for the next three weeks. The body likes to be surprised and stimulated.

HOW TO USE THE OILS

Bath-time

After body brushing in the way described in Step 6, shake between six to ten drops of essential oil (not the massage oil) into the bath. Lie there, if possible, for about 15 minutes, breathing deeply and letting the concentrated oil do its work. As you lie in the bath, knead and pummel the cellulite-heavy areas. You will soon get to know which these are.

Time for a massage

After getting out of the bath and drying yourself, rub some of the diluted oil into each thigh and the buttocks, paying particular attention to the cellulite areas. Make sure you massage the oil in well (see Step 8 for how to do this). The oils will take about ten minutes to be absorbed completely, and there will be no residual 'oiliness' on your skin after this time. The oils should not spoil or stain clothes if you rub them in sufficiently.

Using an oil burner

You can also burn oils to inhale the fragrance. Oil burners can be bought in most craft shops and fill the air with a wonderful fragrance that has potent de-stressing qualities. Six drops of essential oil in water are all you need to release the fragrance. This can be done whenever you don't have time for a bath, and should be done as often as you can.

WHEN AND HOW OFTEN?

It is best to perform the anti-cellulite treatments either first thing in the morning or, if you don't have time, then in the early evening. Don't do it last thing at night, not because it is dangerous but because the combination of skin brushing, bath and massage will probably keep you awake as the overall effect is extremely stimulating.

At first you should do the body brushing, aromatherapy and massage every day. Then, after about three or four weeks, use the massage oils every other day. When most of the cellulite has dispersed – and you will know this by your new sleek outline and lack of dimples – use the body brush plus the oils just once or twice a week.

As you progress with the treatment you will probably notice that previously hard areas of thigh and buttock have become soft and flabby. Now, you may think that flab is as bad as cellulite, but actually it's not. This kind of flab is a temporary condition brought about when the fatty cells are emptied of their excess water content. Brisk massage and exercise, plus continued use of the aromatherapy oils, will soon tone up flab.

A WORD OF ADVICE: The longer the cellulite has been left, the more difficult it is to get rid of it. So be patient – don't expect everything to happen all at once.

GOING TO A THERAPIST

Women who have huge amounts of cellulite, or fear they may lack the willpower and motivation to give themselves regular treatments, may be better off going to a qualified therapist who has proven successful in treating cellulite.

When you book up an aromatherapist, ask her to give you names of people who have already been treated and speak to them. No reputable therapist will mind putting you in touch with grateful clients – in fact, very many aromatherapists never advertise but get new customers simply by word of mouth.

When speaking to women who have been successfully treated ask how long it took, what it cost and how the treatment progressed. Then if you feel satisfied, book up six sessions. For most people, this should be enough to get rid of the problem. You will usually be advised to have two treatments a week – they are more effective when coming close together.

Usually the first treatment will consist of a consultation where the therapist will ask important questions about your general health. The actual therapy sessions will consist of a vigorous massage session lasting for about half an hour. If the cellulite is really bad or deep, this massage may hurt. A therapist who has been trained in lymphatic drainage massage will really dig in. You will know when she reaches the cellulite points as there may be a moment of sharp pain. During the initial sessions, you may find your legs are covered in bruises afterwards.

Remember that drastic changes will be taking place inside your body as the cellulite disperses and these may be accompanied by insomnia, outbreaks of spots, a slight fluctuation in menstrual patterns, mood changes and negative feelings. You may also get colds, flu and headaches. But don't worry. These are all signs of toxic matter clearing itself out of your system.

The worse the cellulite, the more dramatic the changes will be, but all the nasty side effects will disappear before long. As the treatments proceed, you will feel and become a quite different person. Your body image and self esteem will be raised, and you will notice higher energy levels as the toxins are released from your system.

Note: Although aromatherapy oils are extremely effective at getting rid of cellulite, they will not work unless you also stick to the diet. There is not much point in going to all the trouble and expense of aromatherapy treatments if you continue to smoke, drink and eat junk food, for as fast as you are getting rid of accumulated toxic wastes, new ones are entering the body.

STEP 8
MASSAGE
Get hands on with lymphatic drainage massage

Like aromatherapy, massage was for many years regarded as simply a beauty treatment indulged in by the idle rich. It has also had the rather unfortunate association with sleazy sex parlours. Now it is known that the right kind of massage can have a dramatic effect on the body.

Massage is another very important ingredient of any successful cellulite-removing regime.

TYPES OF MASSAGE

A good type of massage for cellulite areas is **kneading**. For this you have to pretend you are kneading a loaf of bread as you pick up the flesh and squeeze it, applying as much pressure as you can. It is rather like pinching huge areas of flesh (see diagram).

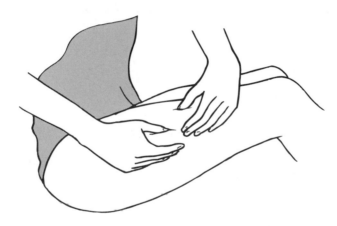

After doing this, you can go back and pinch up the flesh in the very worst of the cellulite areas. You will soon get to know which these are.

Another useful movement for cellulite sufferers is **rolling**. Here, you pick up about an inch of flesh on the thigh and roll it to break down the lumpy deposits.

GET TO KNOW YOUR CELLULITE

After a while you will get to know which areas contain the most cellulite. They will feel ridgy, hard and grainy and you will experience a ripply sensation as you learn to apply more pressure. Long-ingrained cellulite will feel like rows of chipolatas when you massage. These are the areas to concentrate on as the cellulite will need a lot of encouragement to go. Whenever you are massaging your thigh and come across an area which feels particularly tender you can be sure this is where the cellulite is at its worst.

Once you feel you have got to know your cellulite, you can dig at it with your thumb using as much pressure as you are able to do. Any kind of kneading and pinching and pounding will only do good.

Make sure you knead and pound the lumpy areas when you are lying in the bath, especially if you have shaken in a few drops of essential oils. You can also knead and wring the spare flesh at any time of day – whenever you have a few moments of privacy.

A WORD OF WISDOM: When you pummel away at the lumpy areas don't do it with hatred. Very many women – myself included for a long time – feel only disgust when they look down at their thighs and start hating their legs.

When massaging, you should treat your thighs with loving care, reminding yourself that you are doing your very best for them to enable them to lose the rubbish the fat cells have held for so long.

WHEN AND HOW OFTEN?

It is the regularity of massage which makes the difference. Occasional pummelling and kneading is not enough. At first when cellulite is very bad you should make sure you do it every single day. The order is this:

1 Body brushing (see Step 6).

2 A bath with one to six drops of essential oil added (see Step 7).

3 Massaging in the oils (see Step 7 for preparing massage oils). After you get out of the bath, dry yourself. Then pour a little massage oil into the palms of your hands and rub it slightly in. You should never pour any oils directly onto your skin. Then with long stroking movements start at the ankle and work up to the knee and thigh. Use both hands and make sure the movements are gentle but firm. This type of massage encourages circulation and can stimulate blood flow.

Next, rub the massage oil into the thighs and buttocks, paying particular attention to the cellulite areas. Make sure you massage the oil in well – you can use either the kneading or rolling techniques. Then rub a small amount of oil over the stomach to increase detoxification.

The timing of the massage is also important. You probably won't have time to do it properly first thing in the morning and you should not do it last thing at night as the whole exercise can be far too stimulating. So the optimum time is early evening, before supper. If you can get into the habit of performing the massage at this time you will definitely have renewed energy for the evening and you will not be tempted to fill yourself up on snacks and junk foods.

SHOULD YOU ASK FOR HELP?

I have strong doubts about asking people for help. Mostly, people are encouraged to massage each other for sexual or intimate reasons and with cellulite removal this is the last thing on your mind. You are carrying out a self-help medical treatment not indulging in sexual foreplay. For this reason, I would say that it is not a good idea for a husband, boyfriend or lover to try to help you get rid of your cellulite. For one thing, most of them don't care a hoot whether you have cellulite or not, and for another, the intimate kind of stroking needed could soon take a sexual turn. Having said this, it can be difficult to apply the kind of pressure needed on the backs of the thighs yourself. So, if you can persuade somebody to do it for you – with firmness and kindness so it does not hurt – then this will speed up results.

GOING TO A THERAPIST

If you are considering going to a professional, make sure you choose somebody who is qualified to practise both aromatherapy and lymphatic drainage. It is important to ask about lymphatic drainage because this will be your clue that the therapist really can help you. If you get a confused silence on the end of the phone when you ask about this kind of massage, then don't book her up. Also ask, of course, about the nutritional aspects as no massage alone, however tough, can disperse cellulite. It is essential your therapist understands exactly what cellulite is.

WHAT IS LYMPHATIC DRAINAGE MASSAGE – AND HOW CAN IT HELP?

Lymphatic drainage massage is the type of massage most often used in anti-cellulite treatments. This is a very hard, tough type of massage which pummels and kneads away at the cellulite deposits at the same type as activating the lymph nodes. A masseuse does this by pressing on the lymph points all over your body and applying pressure to them. Although you would probably need to go to a professional to get a proper lymphatic drainage, you can easily learn for yourself where the main lymph nodes are and press these after you have finished the kneading and pounding massage.

Waging War on Cellulite Yourself

The diagram below shows where the main lymph nodes are – under the armpits, in the thoracic duct between the breasts, in the lumbar region, behind the knees. It won't take long to learn where these are and touching them will definitely help the lymphatic system to get working properly again.

Some people find that when the body is really loaded with toxic and waste matter the lymph nodes feel tender. If this is the case with you, don't give up, but keep applying gentle pressure until

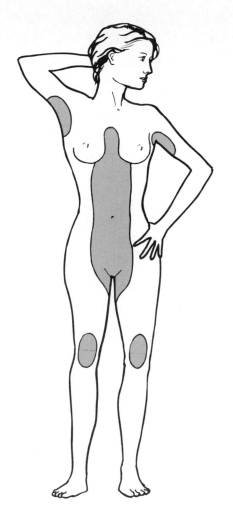

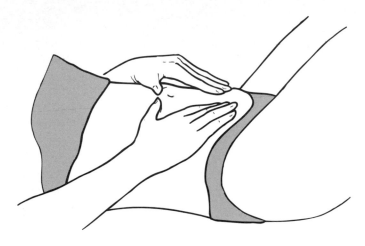

the tenderness ceases. As you carry on with the regime, you will find that the lymph nodes become less tender. Tenderness in these regions means that there is a blockage and it may take time for this to be released.

Most professionals finish up stroking the abdomen gently in circular movements (see diagram). This aids the digestive system and also helps waste products to disperse. It is easy enough to do this for yourself using a tiny trace of oil. Make sure the movements are extremely gentle here.

Going to a Therapist

A professional lymphatic drainage massage will usually take between half and three-quarters of an hour. The therapist will concentrate on only the cellulite areas and the lymphatic points. She will not usually give you a general massage. You can of course ask for a general massage, but this is a different kind of treatment.

The advantage of going to a therapist is that an objective check will be kept on your progress, but don't imagine that all is lost if you cannot find anybody suitable in your area. Once you have the information at your finger-tips and can understand exactly what cellulite is and what is needed to remove it, you can effectively become your own therapist.

TIP: Lymphatic drainage massage can be very hard and tough, and you may feel slightly faint if you get up instantly. If you are doing your own massage, take a tip from the professionals and lie down for a little while after you have finished. I can guarantee you will feel quite wonderful when you get up.

MASSAGE AND STRESS

Anything which helps remove stress, such as massage, is to be recommended. The less tense and anxious you are, the less cellulite will be formed. This is not just some airy-fairy notion but a scientifically acknowledged fact. When the mind is tense and anxious, extra stress hormones (adrenalin) are released into the system and stay there. The more chronic the stress, the greater the release of adrenalin and the greater, eventually, the build-up of toxic wastes.

Digestion, elimination and circulation are all adversely affected by mental stress. We are only just learning – or appreciating – how closely linked the mind and body are, and how intimately the feedback principle operates. Whatever affects the mind will soon reverberate in the body, and vice versa. Massage is a potent means of unstressing the system and thus counteracting the production of excess adrenalin.

As we know, the formation of cellulite is basically an elimination problem, so anything which helps body systems to return to normal will also aid reduction of these wastes.

> **TIP:** You should practise deep breathing for relaxation whenever you have the opportunity, such as when relaxing in the bath. You do it like this. Put both hands on your stomach and as you breathe in, inflate the abdomen. Breathe out slowly, letting the abdomen go back in. Repeat this whenever you think of it. This helps more oxygen get into the system and improves circulation.

A FINAL WORD

One of the benefits of massage is that, after you have been cosseting and caring for your body on the outside this way, you feel much less like putting rubbish into the inside. By massaging yourself you learn to respect your body both inside and out.

You will notice other benefits from regular massage with essential oils. Your skin and clothes will become delicately impregnated with the fragrance of the oils and also your skin will become softer and smoother. You are likely to have far fewer headaches, to feel less irritable and touchy and less stressed generally.

STEP 9
EXERCISE
Time to tone up and get the circulation moving

This is a highly recommended, but optional extra in any cellulite-banishing regime. Exercise can be very effective once you have managed to get rid of the worst of the cellulite and need to tone up the muscles. But there is not much point in embarking on rigorous exercise programmes while you have large areas of cellulite on your thighs. Although the condition is caused by a sedentary lifestyle, vigorous exercise will not make the slightest bit of difference to cellulite deposits that are already there.

A SEDENTARY LIFESTYLE

The vast majority of women who suffer from cellulite are couch potatoes – as well as eating self-indulgently, they never take exercise.

Women who are very active, eat a whole food diet and abstain from alcohol, cigarettes and caffeine will rarely get cellulite. These days, very many women have jobs that necessitate sitting at a desk all day long. Prolonged inactivity of this kind can cut off circulation. When treating cellulite, therapists often notice that cellulite deposits are at their most intractable where the legs meet the chair edge – at the place where circulation is cut off most.

Prolonged physical inactivity leads to an increasingly sluggish circulation, making it even harder for the blood and lymphatic system to get rid of waste materials and send life-giving oxygen round the system.

THE BEST TYPES OF EXERCISE

Many forms of exercise could make cellulite worse, particularly anything that includes jumping up and down or pounding, such as jogging, jazz dancing, aerobics or California-stretch-type exercises. These are emphatically NOT recommended for cellulite removal.

They tend to put extra pressure on the joints and encourage the cellulite to harden and become even more impacted.

The best type of exercise is both gentle and brisk at the same time, such as **walking** or **swimming**. Swimming is, in fact, excellent for cellulite sufferers as it exercises the legs without putting any undue strain on the joints.

Although **yoga** classes will help to put a long-misused body back into alignment, the movements are too slow and sustained to be of enormous help in muscle toning. Yoga positions will certainly help you to find you out where the cellulite-laden areas are, and enable you to realize where stiffness and lack of suppleness lie, but they are not specifically designed to firm up the flab left when cellulite makes its exit.

The good thing about yoga positions, or *asanas* as they are known, is that by doing them – or at least attempting them – you get to know and respect your own body. The other valuable aspect of yoga is that it is not harmful in any way, as perhaps aerobics might be.

WILL MY FLAB EVER GO?

Very often, women who have been on a rigorous anti-cellulite regime find that their legs become flabby and lacking in tone. This is often a temporary condition and can be likened to when you have just had a baby. The minute the baby is born, your stomach is flabby and stretched, like an empty sack. But after a very few weeks it tightens back up again and becomes flat, especially if you do the right kind of exercises to help yourself get back in shape.

Exactly the same process happens with cellulite removal. If the cellulite has been there for a very long time, it will leave a certain amount of flab when it finally goes. Because once cellulite starts to disperse everything can happen very quickly – far too quickly for the skin to stay tight. Don't panic though. Before long the skin will start to 'fit' of its own accord.

WHEN SHOULD I START?

The time to embark on exercise is once the worst of the cellulite has gone. As soon as you begin the anti-cellulite regime you should make up your mind to become as physically active as possible. This means walking instead of taking the bus and going for a swim whenever possible. Any gentle, rhythmic form of exercise will help keep circulation moving which is what you are aiming at.

Once you are left with residual flab, after the worst of the cellulite has made its exit, you can do the tried and tested bicycling in the air, copy somebody who does routines on breakfast television or book keep-fit and conditioning classes at a local gym. Local-authority-run keep-fit and conditioning classes are extremely cheap and usually very good.

A WORD OF ADVICE Never attempt a vigorous work-out if you have been completely sedentary for years on end. This is as much of a shock to the system as a drastically altered diet and the body may not be able to cope.

HOW OFTEN?

After you have completed the anti-cellulite plan in this book, your body and general health will be far better than before and you will probably feel much more like doing exercise. To be effective any exercise has to be regular and you will never keep it up unless you enjoy it. You should walk or swim at least three times a week and, ideally, go to keep-fit classes twice a week. Exercise experts have worked out that in order to do any good, your chosen form of exercise should be practised at least three times a week for at least twenty minutes a time. Any less and you may as well not bother.

A FINAL WORD

If you get rid of the cellulite first, by being conscientious about the plan outlined in this book, and then you complete the good work by the right kind of exercise, you will – I promise you – be rewarded by the kind of figure and good health you had never previously dreamed possible.

It happened to me. And if I, as a lifelong exercise-hater and self-indulgent soul, can get rid of cellulite after more than 20 years, so can you.

STEP 10

KEEP IT UP!
And win the war against cellulite – for good

Cellulite is always liable to come back, much as dust is always trying to settle on household objects, and tarnish on silver and brass. You can only keep it away by constant vigilance. That is the uncomfortable but true fact of life about cellulite.

HOW CAN I PREVENT MY CELLULITE FROM COMING BACK?

To prevent the lumps and bumps from returning, the four ingredients of the anti-cellulite plan you *have to* keep up are: diet, dry skin brushing, massage and exercise.

The anti-cellulite diet has to be a diet for life otherwise your cellulite will reappear and all your hard work will be wasted. Remember that cellulite is always trying to return and take up residence again at the slightest provocation. Of course, there is no harm in the occasional indulgence in an ice-cream, a cream cake or lasagne, but these should never again become a staple part of your diet. If you have a propensity to cellulite then diet is essential for you.

Dry skin brushing should be built into your everyday life if you want to stop cellulite coming back. Keep it away by skin brushing once or twice a week.

You can also help prevent cellulite from coming back by having the occasional **massage**. This will help keep the lymphatic system working properly as well as reducing stress – something that is highly recommended because stress plays a major role in the development of cellulite.

Finally, you should **exercise** on a regular basis to keep the lumps and bumps at bay – exercise experts recommend at least three times a week for at least twenty minutes. As we have seen, one of the main causes of the formation of cellulite is a sedentary lifestyle, which in turn means that circulation is likely to be poor. So exercise is an extremely important step in helping to prevent cellulite by keeping the circulation moving.

A FINAL WORD

The strength of mind needed to combat cellulite successfully should never be over-estimated. I know from personal experience that you have to be single-minded when deciding to banish cellulite. Like an unwelcome guest, it never wants to go, and it will take up permanent squatter's rights in your body whenever it can. You just have to regard it in the same way as household dust and dirt – something you must continually struggle to keep down.

This book is for all those women who have been made miserable by dimpled bulges on their thighs, buttocks and upper arms – bulges they thought they would have to put up with for all their lives.

But if you undertake this 10-step plan, you will soon know that cellulite is not only avoidable – but it is treatable and removable.

You'll not only feel and look far better without the cellulite deposits, your general health will improve as well.

All I can say is – there is no comparison between life with cellulite and life without it.

BIBLIOGRAPHY

Campion, Kitty: *A Woman's Herbal*, Century, 1987

Davies, Dr Stephen and Stewart, Dr Alan: *Nutritional Medicine*, Pan, 1987

Davis, Patricia: *Aromatherapy: An A–Z*, C. W. Daniel, 1988

Gray, Dr Robert: *The Colon Health Handbook*, Rockridge Publishing Company, California, 1983

Hepper, Camilla: *Herbal Cosmetics*, Thorsons, 1987

Kenton, Leslie: *The Joy of Beauty*, Century, 1983

Kenton, Leslie and Kenton, Susannah: *Raw Energy Recipes*, Century, 1985

Maxwell-Hudson, Clare: *The Complete Book of Massage*, Dorling Kindersley, 1988

Maxwell-Hudson, Clare: *Your Health and Beauty Book*, Macdonald, 1979

Maxwell-Hudson, Clare: *The Natural Beauty Book*, Macdonald, 1983

Ryman, Danièle: *The Aromatherapy Handbook*, Century, 1984

Soltanoff, Dr Jack: *Natural Healing*, Warner Books (USA), 1988

Tisserand, Robert: *The Art of Aromatherapy*, C. W. Daniel, 1977

Tisserand, Robert: *Aromatherapy for Everyone*, Penguin, 1988

Valnet, Dr Jean: *The Practice of Aromatherapy*, C. W. Daniel, 1982

West, Ouida: *The Magic of Massage*, Century, 1983

Wright, Brian: *Cleansing the Colon*, Green Press, 1987

Wright, Celia: *The Wright Diet*, Piatkus, 1986

USEFUL ADDRESSES

Aromatherapy courses
The Academy of Aromatherapy and Massage
50 Cow Wynd
Falkirk
Sterlingshire FK1 1PU
Tel: 01324 612 658

The International Federation of Aromatherapy (IFA)
Stamford House
2/4 Chiswick High Road
London W4 1TH
Tel: 020 8742 2605

Aromatherapy Organizations Council
PO Box 19834
London SE25 6WS
Tel: 020 8251 7912

Aromatherapy Oils (mail order)
Bodytreats International
15 Approach Road
Raynes Park
London SW20 8BA
Tel: 020 8543 7633

Micheline Arcier
 Aromatherapy oils and treatments
7 William Street
London SW1
Tel: 020 7235 3545

Neal's Yard Apothecary
Neal's Yard
Covent Garden
London WC2
Tel: 020 7379 7222

The Nutri Centre
7 Park Crescent
London W1N 3HE
020 7436 5122

Body brushes
Simply Nature
Old Factory Buildings
Unit 7
Battenhurst Rd
Stonegate
East Sussex TN5 7DU
01580 201687

Nutri Centre, as above.

Sources of Help
The Alternative Medicine Clinic
Sally Gilbert Wilson
56 Harley House
Marylebone Road
London NW1 5HL
Tel: 020 7486 8087

Nutritional Information
For advice on detoxifying and cleansing diets, contact the sources
listed above.

Massage Courses

The Clare Maxwell-Hudson School of Massage

PO Box 457

London NW2 4BR

Tel: 020 8450 6494

Note: please enclose large s.a.e. when writing to any of these addresses.